AIDS TO ETHICS AND PROFESSIONAL
CONDUCT FOR
STUDENT RADIOLOGIC TECHNOLOGISTS

AIDS TO ETHICS AND PROFESSIONAL CONDUCT FOR STUDENT RADIOLOGIC TECHNOLOGISTS

Second Edition — Fifth Printing

By

JAMES OHNYSTY
R.T.(A.R.R.T.), C.S.R.T.

Department of Radiology
Saint Francis Hospital
Colorado Springs, Colorado

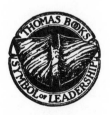

CHARLES C THOMAS • PUBLISHER
Springfield • Illinois • U.S.A.

Published and Distributed Throughout the World by

CHARLES C THOMAS • PUBLISHER

BANNERSTONE HOUSE

301-327 East Lawrence Avenue, Springfield, Illinois, U.S.A.

© *1964 and 1968, by* CHARLES C THOMAS • PUBLISHER

ISBN 0-398-01419-1

Library of Congress Catalog Card Number. 68-18302

First Edition, 1964

Second Edition, 1968

Second Edition, Second Printing, 1970

Second Edition, Third Printing, 1972

Second Edition, Fourth Printing, 1974

Second Edition, Fifth Printing, 1979

Printed in the United States of America

N-1

To the future generation of radiologic technologists; may their education be less difficult to obtain than mine.

FOREWORD

THAT first day, the students walk into a radiology department
and are confused by a new world—a special field of medicine.
Here they will learn to apply themselves to their utmost to contribute in some small way to the healing of the sick. The morning
of that first day will be imbedded as a memory in their minds
for a lifetime. That sudden exposure to terminology and ideas
particular to the study of x-rays and their application to radiography receives most of the students' attention. Many texts are
available for the students to study in the various courses presented
in radiologic technology. In all of these studies, however, attention is focused on theory and technical work; and a very important
subject is overlooked.

Before engaging in the technical work of radiography and concentrating on producing a high standard of radiogram, one must
meet the all-important "patient." Somehow, the confidence and
cooperation of the patient must be gained so that a quality radiogram can be produced. The first impression that the students
present to the patients, to the patients' physicians, to the instructors, and to the radiologists must be favorable. This impression can only come because of understanding, tactfulness, and
efficiency; these qualities are acquired through thorough training.

There are many graduate technologists who work efficiently,
produce excellent radiograms and appear as ideal workers but
in other ways are a failure. They are failures in the minds of
the patients because they have not provided a basic but very necessary psychological need. They must make the patients feel that
they sincerely want to help them get well and that, to them, it
is not "just a job." The patients must be made to feel like who
they really are, "Mrs. Jane Doe" or "Mr. Sam Smith," not a mere
bed number, or Dr. So-and-so's patient, or a broken leg! The
attitude displayed by the technologists during the patients' very
trying times will be remembered for a long time; and, from this,

will be formed an opinion not only of the technologists, but of the department and also the institution.

"Ethics and professional conduct" contribute to the growth and progress of the whole medical profession and increases contributions to the future of mankind.

JAMES OHNYSTY

PREFACE TO SECOND EDITION

THE revision of *Aids to Ethics and Professional Conduct for Student Radiologic Technologists* was undertaken because of two specific reasons—the response to the first edition and the increasing complexity of the psychology of the human mind as we encounter it in our profession. Your opinions and comments were appreciated by the publisher and this author. Your response indicated that a revised, improved and expanded course in "ethics and professional conduct" is needed by one of the fastest growing professions in this paramedical field.

Our profession of radiologic technology is growing by leaps and bounds and many of us who are concerned with the educational program are viewing aggressive, aspiring, young people grappling with the basics of our profession. We cannot overlook the fact that giving our students some fundamental knowledge in anatomy and the scientific principles is not enough. We cannot overlook the need to feel empathy and compassion for our sick and needy fellow man. If we fail to motivate that feeling and the earnest desire within our students to help our fellow man, we will have created the equivalent of human robots. These students will do all forms of calculations and present us with technical results, but they will lack the fundamental emotional human kindness required when working with people. The acceptable norms of our society in a restless world are undergoing constant changes. The youth of today are the leaders of tomorrow and will pave the destiny of the civilized world. The attitudes and ideals of our youth are the important qualities that we must preserve, and we must try to channel their energy towards lessening man's inhumanity to man.

Let us review the changes that have taken place in the field of radiologic technology. We should not look back at the changes of the last decade, but look at the vast changes that have occurred within the very short period of the last five years. These changes and demands are so rapid and overwhelming that procedures and principles recently used are becoming rapidly outmoded and obsolete for meeting the demands of the present, much less the future.

In the past, radiologic technology, better known to us of the older generations as x-ray technology, was a little known field that literally everyone took a swing at. The concensus of opinion established in many circles was that x-ray work did not require any particular talent. It seems the general idea of the past was that you picked up a few basic ideas in how to operate the machines, how to position a certain part of the anatomy on top of a film, and by trial and error you obtained a reasonably diagnostic radiogram.

This whole idea evolved around x-ray technology until a few devoted, skilled, dedicated technologists, through determined efforts, organized a program of education. Their persistent efforts, plus the growing demands of the rapidly advancing field of radiology in medicine, developed radiologic technology into one of the fastest growing and demanding paramedical fields.

Invariably whenever a group expands too rapidly, be it a society or a nation, many loose ends are left behind unattended, and there are weaknesses in the structure. One of these weaknesses was ethics and professional conduct, which every individual must train himself to possess if he is to be a successful radiologic technologist. Success is measured not only by the degree of technical skills and accomplishments, but also the degree to which you fulfill the emotional needs of your patient.

The subject material of this book is as diversified and controversial as the sum total of each of you who read it. Many of you will not agree with some views found in this book. These may not coincide with your general ideas of what you would do or how you have met the challenge of these particular problems in the past. However, you are challenged to read, to evaluate, and to debate the problems of ethics and professional conduct within our profession.

Technologists are made; they are not born. Only radiologic technologists can perpetuate the profession and educate future technologists. We must strive to progress not only in our technical skills but in our sense of values, our duties and our obligations. Radiologic technology must not be simply a means to material gains, but a work of love and devotion for the progress of medicine in the preservation of human life.

The author takes this opportunity to thank the many colleagues from ocean to ocean, from border to border, and from the various countries of the free world for contributing their opinions and ideas. Regardless of what your opinion was, it was helpful in the compilation of this second edition.

Many people gave inspiring ideas in the preparation of this edition. One of the chief contributors to this book and my severest critic is my "better half," who offered constructive opinions, criticisms and encouragement in equal measures. My sincere appreciation to V'Lee Sawyer, the typist and editing advisor, who so cheerfully and efficiently perused my notes. Grateful appreciation is acknowledged to the publisher for advice and encouragement.

J. O.

PREFACE TO FIRST EDITION

AFTER some years of teaching, having been confronted with many problems of ethics and conduct in training radiologic technologists, it was decided to do some research on the topic. Reading through volumes of books and medical journals, the author found himself little further ahead than when he started. Of course, there were a great number of rules and regulations that one must follow; but none gave examples or practical reasons "why." So, after pondering over the subject, placing himself in the student's situation, he remembered that he, himself, had to learn through experience by trial and error. Nowhere was there any material to guide him on how to deal with a particular type of patient or a given situation. There were a number of rules with many "do's" and "don'ts" but never "why" or "where." How can an inquisitive and inexperienced mind visualize the problems that it will be confronted by?

Upon consulting some of the key instructors across the country, the author found that there is no one book on ethics and conduct. This particular phase of training has been passed over with only relatively little thought and discussion. No one, yet, seems to have realized just how "apparent" thorough moral training is in the work of a professional person, and how aware the patient is of it. Too long we have left the development of professional conduct and ethics to the individual's own discretion through trial and error; too many times we have harmed the patient and not been aware of it; too many times we have lowered the standard of our profession by our own lack of tact and understanding. Have you any idea of the unpleasant memories the patient will retain? Perhaps we succeeded in getting a good radiogram, but what of our attitude and manners to the patient as an "individual?"

Sitting back and thinking this problem through, it was realized that this is one of the major problems in our profession and perhaps in other medical professions. In all fairness to the future generations of Radiologic Technologists, something had to be done. We need more than just cold, hard rules. We need examples and possible solutions for the students to use in motivating them to think out these problems and realize the importance of them. If we are to have our students learn and progress as an asset to themselves and our profession, then we must stop making errors without realizing just how serious they are.

A project such as this was not easy to accomplish or to assemble for presentation as a learning manual. The material herein comes from notes gathered over a period of years; a great deal of it comes from the author's own personal trials and tribulations, some not easily forgotten. Chiefly, though, it was derived from observing students and sitting down with them to solve the problems at hand. This text is not intended as a set of rules and regulations for the students to study, or for the instructors to present. On the contrary, the purpose in compiling this book is to have the instructor and the students discuss and arrive at a comparable solution, should they be faced with similar problems. This type of study is limitless and would lead into psychology from birth to death with theories illimitable as to the whys and wherefores of human reactions. The basic motive is to present some major problems that confront radiologic technology students each day and to suggest ways of dealing with them.

Undoubtedly, there will be many persons who will not agree with these suggestions or ideas; even so, this will have accomplished a major victory—for it will have motivated you, the reader, to discuss and think about these problems. It is felt that if you become more interested in our fellow man, then, together, we will have started a worthwhile project.

The author's wife, by giving viewpoints from the patient side plus much constructive criticism, was his strongest supporter in this project. Sincere appreciation is expressed to his superiors, Drs. V. L. Bolton and C. W. Partington, who supported this project, and to V'Lee Sawyer, who graciously waded through the handwritten notes and typed the manuscript.

J. O.

CONTENTS

[xiv]

AIDS TO ETHICS AND PROFESSIONAL
CONDUCT FOR
STUDENT RADIOLOGIC TECHNOLOGISTS

CHAPTER I

PERSONALITY AND ATTITUDES REQUIREMENTS

M AN'S greatest challenge is "life" itself. As he surveys his environment and discerns that rapid, revolutionary changes are constantly being made, he strives to also achieve some measure of happiness and material wealth. Rare is the man who feels he has achieved his full measure of life and its riches.

Regardless of the type of life that man plans for himself, be it material wealth, the spiritual satisfaction of helping others, or the achievement of fame and power to any degree, there exists one unchangeable factor. Regardless of any man's power on earth, this factor is that he is not immortal. Naturally, in the spirit and preoccupation of living, man seldom admits this until suddenly or insidiously his life is threatened. Whenever man's health is in question, a small pang of fear gnaws its way into the conscious mind with the realization that he is vulnerable. Though he is an intellectually superior being, he is physically weak, because this active, intelligent human body can be stilled in a split second!

When you have a financial problem, you visit with your banker or credit consultant. When you have problems with your automobile, you visit your car dealer or service station. When you have a problem with your health, you visit the key individual of the medical profession, your physician.

The field of modern medicine is a complicated organization composed of precision teams, including various paramedical professions, all working for one common goal—to preserve, maintain or restore the health of man. Radiologic technologists comprise one small, important team that plays a very essential part in the practice of the art and science of medicine.

Any individual who is about to embark on a medical or paramedical career, regardless of the specialty, must possess one basic and essential characteristic quality. He must sincerely desire to help his fellow man. He must want to devote his knowledge, his time and his concentrated effort to help other people. With this basic foundation, this requirement of attitude, he can develop all of the other qualities. He must develop numerous qualities in order to achieve the utmost success in his undertaking of a medical profession.

Let us now pursue a classified and detailed study of the complicated qualities one must develop and possess to achieve some measure of success in the art of "communication." As you come in contact with patients, colleagues, instructors, physicians, and others, you must emanate the attitudes becoming to your status as a student. As you grow and develop with the profession, you must accept the responsibilities that come to you and fulfill your obligations with the dignity becoming to a professional individual.

Personality and Attitudes

You are about to embark on a new phase of your life, in a profession laden with more responsibility than you have ever assumed or even imagined. Responsibility cannot be stressed sufficiently for you to fully realize its scope, and you will be faced with it constantly as you go about your daily duties. Your greatest responsibilities are to yourself and the aims and ideals of your profession as set up by individuals with foresight and devotion in the Code of Ethics of the American Registry of Radiologic Technologists. If you can fulfill these obligations and those as set down in "The X-Ray Technician's Pledge," you will have served well your patient, the physicians and the institution.

Together let us review some of the personality and attitudes requirements for anyone pursuing a medical profession. Let us reminisce for a few moments and try to remember what prompted you to undertake this profession. No doubt there are several reasons, and together they formed a pattern that influenced your final decision. There may be numerous reasons why you decided to undertake radiologic technology. It could have been that you could not afford to go to college and were influenced by your family to take this course and become self-supporting in two years. It could have been that possibly your high-school grades did not qualify you to enroll in college in some specific course. It could have been due to any number of material considerations, or do you perhaps have a greater motivation? Is it possible that because of some personal experience or influence in your child-hood, possibly an experience in the hospital, that you were in-spired to contribute yourself to helping others? Do you wish to become a member of a team of professional people striving to maintain or restore the health of their fellow man? Do you need to fulfill an inner desire that will only be satisfied from the knowl-edge that you have helped someone less fortunate? These are some of the basic reasons that should have motivated you for entering the profession of radiologic technology. If you practice your pro-fession sincerely and faithfully, you can only be a credit to it.

The concensus of opinion by appearances is that a successful man is one who has gained a great deal of material wealth and personal recognition. Material wealth can be calculated in dollars and cents. It may qualify man for social prominence, etc.; but, in a paramedical profession, one rarely captures the society page or becomes a social butterfly. Our rewards will not come socially and perhaps may not be evident to the selfish and shallow individual for they are present in our spiritual satisfaction.

Graduation is not the end of your learning process. Your cer-tificate will not open the door to absolute security so that you can just sit back and coast along through life. Graduation in any profession simply opens the door to greater demands and hard work. Your radiologic technology diploma provides you with the foundation upon which to build your profession and fulfill its aims and objectives.

Definite guidelines cannot be established for what you must do upon graduation. You may wish to go forth and dedicate your-self to improve your work and expand your knowledge within the profession; use your education in radiologic technology as a stepping stone to further educate yourself and possibly undertake more advanced studies; stabilize yourself financially, or travel in your work. There are many avenues you can follow.

One must understand that study in any branch of medicine and its associated professions is limitless; there is no one set of books that has recorded more than a fraction of what is already known. Medicine is one of the fastest growing professions, and it is believed that we are only scratching the surface within our own profession of radiologic technology. Consequently, graduation is only the key to greater avenues of learning, and we must understand that we are merely amateurs advancing toward the major leagues.

As you read this particular section at the onset of your training, sit back and evaluate the circumstances and the possibilities of this profession. Are your motivations sincere or are they purely personal and only the means to earn a livelihood? You must realize that you will need to contribute yourself to others. Certainly as students, your thoughts are of learning a great deal, passing all of the examinations and finally the Registry Examination. Since we do live in a rocket speed age of progress, we must, even though we may hesitate, set our sights on a goal far beyond our training.

No profession or organization can survive if its members do not strive to elevate its standards and progress with the times. The radiologic technology profession is one of the newly organized paramedical professions. The American Registry of Radiologic Technologists and the American Society of Radiologic Technologists were formed by individuals with ideals and foresight who had a keen interest and faith in the value and urgent need of its organization. It is the personal responsibility of each of us not only to maintain but to continue building our profession. You will need to remember that you have to dedicate yourself to the other man who needs your services, your knowledge and your devotion.

Actually, in any business or profession, you will get out of your work no more than you contribute. If you have studied diligently and developed yourself to the best of your ability and if you are devoted to your profession, you will grow with it. If you are ready to apply yourself—devote yourself and contribute yourself unselfishly—then you have the basic foundation to face the challenge ahead.

It is not the intention to get philosophical and inspire you on the surface, but you should understand that you will be doing serious, meaningful work. Therefore, you must possess an inner fortitude and a set of moral values that are strong enough to sustain you as you pursue this line of work.

Great demands of conduct, personality and attitudes will be made of you, by your patients and by the professional people with whom you come in contact. Perhaps much of the society around us does have the attitude, "live today, for tomorrow never comes." However, we must be creative and build to uphold the existence of mankind itself. The world does not "owe us a living." All that mankind now possesses was built up by the strong men with ideals, foresight, persistence and a set of values.

CHAPTER II

THE SMALL WORLD WITHIN THE HOSPITAL WALLS

As a general rule, life begins and ends in the hospital. You will witness the miracle of birth and the agony of death many times over. You will need to realize that for each there is a purpose, not ours to question.

There are many methods used in the process of sustaining life and restoring body functions. In the sections that follow we shall undertake to discuss the various approaches and means of communication with the patient as we play our part in achieving these goals.

You have no doubt been in the hospital on other occasions. Perhaps you were a patient or visited a friend or relative who was a patient. You may have been impressed by the quiet, yet cheerful, efficient personnel; namely nurses, doctors, technologists, and others with whom you came in contact in the various departments. Perhaps it would be a good idea to take stock of your first impressions and reevaluate them. If you plan to study in this institution and become a part of it, you must look at this new world in its true reality.

The hospital is comparable to an intricate machine in itself. It is a combination of multiple components interdependent upon each other but working together for a common, ultimate goal. The atmosphere and working conditions are different from all others outside the hospital. The patients who are in the hospital are sick, or they think they are or their doctors think they are. They are in the hospital not because they want to be, but because it is imperative if they are to have their health restored.

You are familiar with the society in the outside world and have seen, or perhaps been a part of, the group of people performing different services in the commercial field. These people usually greet you with a cheerful smile, the atmosphere is devoid of tension and the customers are free to choose or reject your type of service as they desire. There is no tension, reluctance or fear involved. In the hospital the customers, who are the patients, may not be in a position to be relaxed and cheerful. They will be worried and apprehensive about their tests, the results of these tests, the success or failure of their treatments or surgery. They will be afraid of the unknown.

The working conditions in a hospital are different in many ways from those existing in our offices, schools, stores, etc. If you work in a department store you will begin your work about nine o'clock and quit at about five. You will probably have two or more coffee breaks and time for lunch; at closing time you pick up your personal belongings and go home. Hospital work cannot be turned on and off at specified times. People do not get sick at appointed hours; on the contrary there may be a greater need for your services at two in the morning rather than two in the afternoon. The hospital operates twenty-four hours a day, seven days a week, every week of the year, Sundays and holidays included. It is impossible to close its doors on weekends or holidays.

Perhaps you would like an example of what conditions you are likely to encounter. It is ten-thirty Saturday night. Suddenly you hear a siren and an ambulance pulls up to the emergency entrance. Two stretchers are brought in; the patients are taken to the emergency room. The resident doctor examines the first patient who has several cuts on his head and is bleeding from the nose and right ear, his arm is evidently broken and severely displaced, he has several abrasions on his chest. A quick preliminary examination by the resident doctor gives him the impression that this patient may have a fractured skull; he may also have a fractured arm plus possible chest injuries. This patient will no doubt require immediate surgery if his condition is such that it may be performed; however, the doctors must know what fractures there are, their exact location and severity.

Now comes your part. The patient may be bleeding internally and could go into shock; emergency measures have been taken to control and prevent this; however, the danger is still great. You have to work quickly and this means *"Quickly."* Remember, there is no time for error or a second chance for you to do repeat radiograms if your first are of unacceptable quality. You must use all of your acquired knowledge with speed and organized efficiency, for, remember, a life may be dependent upon your capabilities. You are part of a team of professional people all with one goal in mind; to save a human life. There is an air of tension; you are under pressure, but you come through because you are a trained, devoted individual with an earnest desire to help others. Yes, this is late at night; the average office worker is home watching television or out for an enjoyable evening with friends. You are working hard mentally, emotionally, and often physically with a purpose; this is what makes you a professional person.

You will often come in contact with patients who are in agonizing pain or others who are emotionally overwrought to the point of delirium. It is at times like these that you need to be levelheaded and provide reassurance and comfort to those who need it. You must see that nothing adds to their agony and, at the same time, try to quiet them. These patients must be made to feel that they can rely on you for help. You must be able to give them a feeling of confidence in you and your work; this can only be so if you are a skilled technologist and have confidence in yourself. You must be able to handle them in such a way that you do not add to their discomforts and fears and they, in turn, will cooperate with you.

CHAPTER III

FIRST IMPRESSIONS OF THE DEPARTMENT OF RADIOLOGY

MOST likely you have been forming impressions during your first week or month of training. These impressions are of the radiologists, the school director, the chief technologist, the instructors, the registered technologists, the other students and the department as a whole. Your impressions may be favorable or they may be confused and doubtful. In this section we will try to explain these people to you so that you will be in a better position to understand them; to form more realistic impressions of them, their relationship to the department and the institution as a whole. Your first impressions are important; they will affect your training and your attitudes towards your training, the school, and the department.

Your first contact with the department personnel was probably the director of the school; this individual perhaps conducted your first interview, told you about the course of study and explained the training program in general. More often the director will be a radiologist or a technologist of several years' experience. You should not form instinctive first impressions too solidly, for you may be quite incorrect in your evaluation. Your relationship with the director of the school is very important throughout your entire training. Let us examine the probabilities of this individual, his attitude and mannerisms.

Director of the School of Radiologic Technology

The medical director of the school, who is the radiologist, has a grave and important responsibility to you as an individual. He is aware, in this capacity, that his responsibility is to train students to become the best possible technologists. The training he presents to you in every aspect, from the technical knowledge and skills to the ethical conduct and attitudes, will depend largely upon his guidance. The incentive he promotes in you is important, for he understands that the future of the profession will depend upon individuals like yourself. You are the potential future of the radiologic profession and must therefore be developed into skilled, professionally devoted technologists. He will need to answer for your success or failure in your training program.

You must understand that you cannot shed all of the responsibilities on the school director for developing you into a technologist. A director will look upon you as a mature adult, who of his own free will has chosen this profession, has come to learn, to master his work to the best of his ability. If you have the initiative, the desire, the will to work day and night, and literally live with this training program, you will learn the maximum in this two-year period.

The training program that the director of the school uses, the curriculum that he will follow will be current as set forth by the curriculum of the American Society of Radiologic Technologists. He has the responsibility of conducting the classes regularly and covering the complete program according to established standards. You must keep in mind that his responsibility is not just to teach you to pass the Registry Examination, but to give you a solid foundation in your training program so that you are capable of advancing with the profession after you graduate. He must give you the impetus to continue learning after graduation and you will quickly realize that learning is a continuous process for the duration of your lifetime.

Your responsibilities to the director of the school are such that you must give him your full cooperation and be eager to learn. He cannot tolerate students who do not maintain an interest in the course, who do not complete their assigned homework, who do not show consistent progress in their training program. He knows that just preparing you to pass the Registry Examination will not sufficiently prepare you to go out into the professional world, and that if you fail as a technologist you will tend to blame your training school for your downfall. You need to be honest with yourself and with him for he is not only your director and instructor, he is also your counselor. He will counsel you in regard to the progress of your training, and whether or not it is satisfactory. He has no time to waste on half-hearted, half-interested students who are trying to slide through training.

School directors have a common goal—to make the best possible technologists out of you, by giving you the best possible training. They realize that some of you will one day be responsible for future training programs. Any inadequacies in your training may be reflected in the students that you may supervise or instruct in the future.

Chief Technologist

Your relationship with the chief technologist is also very important in your training program. The chief technologist has a great deal of responsibility relative to his position. He has to maintain a smoothly running, efficient department; the referring physicians have to be happy with the service of the department to the patients and to them. The radiologists must be satisfied with the work of their technologists. The quality of the radiographic work being done in any department depends upon the skill and supervision of the chief technologist. The students in any work tend to copy and imitate their seniors. If the technologists and instructors know their work, the radiograms will be of high diagnostic quality and the students will be properly technically trained.

There can be only one boss in any department. The senior must assume the responsibility and the students must obey and follow, doing as they are instructed. No chief technologist can command respect if he plays favorites among his students or the other technologists. Everyone must be treated equally on a formal, professional basis. The chief technologist has the responsibility for all sections of the department and for all of the actions of his students and staff; many times he will need to answer to the radiologists and the hospital administration for errors that the students or technologists make. He also knows that your success or failure depends a great deal upon his ability to teach and supervise you in your training.

The chief technologist may be very strict and demanding and

sometimes you may not understand his techniques or ideas. You should realize that he is under the orders of his superiors and works with their approval. If you find it difficult to understand any of the rules or policies, discuss them with your chief technologist or perhaps the director of the school. Do not resist rules and regulations simply because you find them demanding or difficult. If you abide by them, you will come to understand them as you mature and you will appreciate those who made you follow them.

Instructors

If this is a larger training center, your next contacts in the radiology department will be the individual instructors. These people have learned their work beyond the requirements for a staff technologist and are devoted to the teaching of others. They must be learned enough to be able to explain and demonstrate in a manner from which a student can easily learn. Most of these instructors have an educational background beyond the basic radiologic technologists' training level and have certificates in teaching. Theirs is a responsible and difficult task to make qualified professional technologists. "It is a difficult task!" Take advantage of lectures and demonstrations; follow their instruction and try to appreciate their efforts. Dedicated teachers put forth much more effort than is required because they have pride in their work.

Staff Technologists

Staff technologists working in the department have the responsibility of carrying out the technical work to the best of their ability. A large percentage of staff technologists are trained in specific fields of radiologic technology with the capabilities of doing their work accurately, effectively and quickly. The staff technologists will have the responsibility of supervising your practical work and assisting you in developing your technical skills to the level that is required within the department. You need to respect these individuals for their knowledge and skills and learn from them as they guide you.

Religious Orders

If you are a student in a Catholic hospital, your chief technologist or the director of the school may be a sister in a religious order. A sister has all the duties of her position plus several of her own. She has taken certain vows and has numerous daily religious duties. If you are of the Catholic faith you will find her an excellent confidant and advisor. If you are not of the same faith do not suspect that you will always be considered as second best. If the sister has accepted you into training, she is obviously aware of your religious affiliation and respects your right to adhere to the same. She will be equally concerned about you as a student and counsel you if you request it. Freedom of religion is one of the basic freedoms of our nation; practice the one of your choice and respect the rights of others to do the same.

Many students find that they are uneasy in the presence of a sister. This is justified only inasmuch as you will find that their personalities differ from one individual to another like those of anyone else. A sister technologist in charge of a training program is one of the most devoted individuals you can find, relative to training students to the highest caliber of technologists. Their one desire is to devote themselves to their profession and guide you in the best possible way so that you may achieve the highest goals in this field. Do not feel ill at ease when a sister is present; just be assured that she is an understanding individual, even though her attire is different and her rules of conduct are very strict and exacting. The sisters are highly intelligent individuals with a sense of humor, who have a wide expanse of knowledge both in their professional field and their religious calling. You have a great deal to gain by working with these devoted individuals. A sister in the position of chief technologist or director of the school may sometimes appear strict or unreasonable; however, remember that all she has to gain from her students is a group of intelligent, qualified, professional technologists.

Radiologists

Here is a specialized physician, perhaps two or more, whom you have met only briefly. You know that they are physicians who are specialists in the field of radiology, but how will they affect your period of training? Indirectly, they will have a great deal to do with your training and mainly this will come by way of the director of the school or the chief technologist. The presence of a radiologist may make you feel uneasy but remember that they are there to do special procedures and read and diagnose all of the radiograms. They will also present part of the teaching program in giving you classes in the more detailed aspects of anatomy, physiology, and radiography. For the present, respect them for their qualifications and knowledge. They will become aware of you only after you start proving yourselves as good students and potential technologist material. They will guide the teaching program prescribed by the National Society curriculum.

Fellow and Senior Students

Within the department you will observe senior students moving about, busy as beavers, working earnestly and devotedly. These students are intent on their work and studies because they realize the importance of it and their personal responsibilities for doing their best. They are striving to help the patient, to improve in their work, to perfect their techniques so that they are more dependable and the patient will benefit from their services. Some day you may be as efficient as they, and perhaps even better. You have much to learn, and you will work along with these individuals when you reach your junior session of training. The atmosphere in the department must be one of harmony; cooperation with your fellow students and other personnel is imperative. There must be no petty jealousies or bickering among you. Do not try to advance your own position at the expense of someone else.

Fellow colleagues in your class are individuals like yourself, earnestly trying to evaluate this whole profession as they step into a new world of training and responsibility. You will study with them, you will practice with them, you will discuss and debate; try to contribute to and develop a positive class spirit. Treat your fellow colleagues with courtesy and respect. Do not be prejudiced if they catch on to the work and studies more quickly than you. On the other hand, do not belittle those who are slower than you. Be respectful of everyone around you, because taking advantage of anyone—or vice versa—can create havoc and numerous problems within the department. The only solution to such a problem is instant dismissal of the guilty party. The profession can do well without cheats, tattle tales and favor-seekers.

Do not form any strong impressions about your colleagues at this time. They are certain to be having reservations about you and the others and will show up their true personalities in time. As time progresses, with proper guidance from the instructors, you will all be able to adapt your personalities, ideas and opinions to each other and work in unison as a professional team intent on learning and developing your knowledge and skills.

Radiology Department

In general, you have now met all of the professional personnel in an average department. You are slowly becoming a part of this efficient, working team. You will work together studying, learning, researching and advancing yourselves, all for improvement of service to the patients and their physicians. One fact that you must realize is that as you walk into the department of radiology, you are no longer a carefree adolescent; you are expected to behave as a mature adult. You must begin thinking as an adult and a professional individual. Do not start off on the wrong foot by setting your own guidelines and ideas. Be receptive to rules and regulations as predetermined by experienced individuals. Do not start off by being lazy, selfish and attempting to get away with the least possible work— thinking that perhaps you won't get caught at it! Remember that you are low man on the totem pole and as far as the profession of radiologic technology is concerned you are just beginners. If you resent being disciplined, criticized or corrected, then perhaps you may not belong in this demanding program and should reevaluate the choice you have made. Perhaps it would be advisable to be realistic and choose a less demanding, nonprofessional occupation.

Be honest with yourself and the school. Your initial ideas and opinions will change as you come to understand your work, hopefully in a positive direction. You should feel a little humble and appreciative of the people who have to tolerate your errors, spend countless hours instructing and correcting you so that you may become technologists. Show your appreciation by being interested, inquiring and displaying a mature, adult attitude towards the program.

CHAPTER IV

TOUR OF THE HOSPITAL AS A WHOLE UNIT

PAY particular attention to each individual department as a unit and its separate function.

Now that you have enrolled in the school and commenced your studies, you will need to familiarize yourself with the different departments of the hospital. You will be associating with many of the personnel and should know something of their duties and responsibilities.

Administrator

The administrator is responsible for the function of the hospital as a complete unit, and has been trained to be proficient in this capacity. The various department heads consult with the administrator with regard to the individual departmental problems. This individual is extremely busy but will be interested in meeting you and welcoming you to the hospital family. As a student you will have very little contact with the administrator since your school director and chief technologist are your direct superiors and deal with the departmental problems. The administrator should be treated with courtesy and respect on any occasion that you may meet. It will be appreciated and recognized as an indication of your maturity and professional conduct.

Administrative Assistant or Business Manager

This individual is responsible for the purchasing of supplies and equipment for the institution and accounting for all expenses. The chief technologist will have many dealings with him in regard to equipment and supplies for the radiology department. In turn, you will have countless lectures from the chief technologist relative to the expenses within the radiology department. A hospital is a very expensive institution to maintain and the radiographic department is among the most costly. If you are efficient and prudent in your use of supplies and equipment, you can contribute much to the economical function of running the department.

Credit Manager

This department is responsible for issuing regular statements to the patients for their hospital bills and to make individual arrangements for the payment of same.

Personnel Director

The personnel director deals with all of the individual personal problems of the personnel. He does all of the hiring and the firing and is responsible for adequate staffing of all departments. He is called upon to solve many intricate interdepartmental and intradepartmental problems. As a student you will have few dealings with this individual, since most of your problems will be handled through the chief technologist or the school director. In most institutions this department will distribute the payroll and student stipend, pending the policy of the school. All employees must attend meetings when called by the personnel director to discuss changes of policy, etc. Hospital social functions are often handled by this office. You may be called upon to represent your department on committees. Remember that in such instances you represent not only yourself but your department and school. Full support and cooperation will be expected of you.

Admission and Information Department

This is the first contact that the all-important patient has with the hospital. Here he supplies the pertinent personal statistics and information for the hospital records and for the use of the private health insurance companies who deal directly with the hospital. From this office, the patients will be assigned to the departments which provide the services they require. Very often, patients will be directed to the department of radiology for preliminary radiographic examinations before being taken to their assigned rooms. Good communication and relations between this office and the radiology department will expedite having these examinations completed quickly, eliminating inconvenience to the patient. Frequently the admission clerks will come to the radiology department to get information from accident patients while the films are being processed. The departments must co-operate with each other, in order to carry out their respective duties in a quick, efficient manner. Readily you will need to go to the admissions office to get more information about a patient or to submit requisitions or charge slips. Communication and cooperation are essential for efficient service to the patient.

Out-Patient Department

This department takes care of minor treatments, injections and other problems for which the patient does not need to be admitted. These patients are also at times scheduled for radiographic examinations and should be handled quickly and efficiently for the convenience of the patient and the physician. You will have numerous patients coming to you from the Out-Patient Department, and both departments will need to cooperate for the benefit of the patient.

Emergency Room

The emergency department cares for patients who require immediate treatment. Many of these are accident victims who have broken bones, flesh or internal injuries or burns. The majority of these accident victims will require radiographic examinations and this is one service where speed and efficiency are of the utmost importance. These two departments must work together as a team. Life may be dependent upon the combined efficiency of both.

Medical Laboratory

This department is very interdependent with the radiology department. It is divided into subdepartments dealing with the chemistries of the human body. Blood studies, tissue studies, urinalyses, etc., are but a few of the numerous studies. Our respective departments depend upon each other for confirmation of diagnoses. Often a patient is scheduled for both laboratory and x-ray work on the same day and scheduling must not conflict. There will be basic chemistry procedures that you will need to know in order to understand radiographic examinations. In many training schools, it is a required part of the curriculum that students spend some of their time in the medical laboratory.

Surgery Department

Many of your specialized studies will take place in the surgery department. Many surgical procedures require radiographic examinations in order to aid the surgeon. You will become a member of the surgical team doing your share of the work with the radiographic knowledge that you have. Your radiograms will guide the surgeon in the correct and accurate setting of bones and detecting radiographic substances not visible to the naked eye. Technologists must be taught sterile operating room techniques and surgical procedures in addition to knowing their radiographic techniques. This is one area where study is vital, speed and efficiency are imperative and you will have to achieve this proficiency in order to qualify to work in this department.

Many of the departments, built in the past few years, will do specific radiographic procedures which require that the patient be under anesthesia, in the surgery department. In this instance, the nurses and technologists must work together in order for the examination to be successful—in other words, they must have "cooperation."

Pharmacy and Sterile Supply Service

Many drugs are used in the radiology department and you will need to know about them and the radiographic examinations for which they are used. The use of drugs is a very exacting and important procedure. There are many whose names are similar but whose chemical components vary enough to be fatal if the wrong drug is administered. Drugs should be administered by the radiologist but you may be the one responsible for setting them out for him. You must always show the attending physician the drugs that you have set out and make available for him to read and check the labels before they are administered to the patient.

Many drugs are subject to chemical changes if exposed to air or light for several weeks. It is important that you familiarize yourself with the various drugs and the different problems that may be encountered. You should understand what actions are to be taken if certain allergic reactions occur and have the anti-allergic drugs immediately available to be administered by the physician.

Nearly every day new drugs for use in radiology departments are released on the market. It is important that you keep currently informed on all of these drugs and on pertinent information relative to their uses, actions, etc. One word of caution: *Never* administer any drug without first having a written or verbal order from the physician or radiologist. The physician or radiologist must be present in the department at time of administration. Rules and regulations for the administering of drugs will vary from one institution to another and from one state to another. Familiarize yourself with the particular regulations in your institution; your best counsel in this regard would be the chief technologist. These regulations are designed to protect both the patient and the personnel and it is imperative that you adhere to them.

Nursing Service Departments

Each nursing service floor provides care particular to one type of patient. Medical, surgical, pediatric (children), geriatric (aged), and obstetrical nursing, intensive and coronary care nursing are some of the services that are provided in every hospital. You will come in contact with all of these patients coming for different types of radiographic studies. Each of these types of patients requires a different approach and a different method of doing procedures in radiography.

It is important that you be familiar with the policies of each of these individual floors, where to find the rooms and the bed numbering arrangement used in semi-private or ward rooms. If there is cooperation between the nursing staff and the radiology department you should never make a mistake in picking up the wrong patient or returning a patient to the wrong room or bed. Whenever a student leaves the department and enters another department to either get or return a patient, he is in foreign territory, so to speak. Consequently, he will follow the rules and regulations of that department under the administration of the floor supervisor. Even as a student, remember that you must develop your personality to be able to get along with the personnel on the different floors. Your presence, cooperation, your attitudes represent not only you but the school and the department.

One of the stumbling blocks in cooperation between the departments is communication. Even at this particularly early stage of your training, you must understand that the proper and complete relating of orders is imperative. Avoid errors and delays in diagnosis due to improperly or incompletely related orders to the nursing personnel. You must develop a tolerant attitude towards the mistakes of others. If a nurse were to criticize you personally, or your department, you must not get into any verbal disagreement. Be courteous, then relate this particular information to your chief technologist. Let him settle the problem with the nurses, because you do not command the respect to fend for yourself in this rather complicated and touchy situation. The chief technologist will determine the credibility of the criticism and follow through with the proper solution. Since the goal of the two departments involves service to the patient, there must be cooperation between the two in providing their respective services.

Physiotherapy Department

The physiotherapy department devotes itself to the rehabilitation of paralyzed and debilitated patients. Their disabilities are due to injuries or disease. Often these injuries are first determined through radiography, and progress of the physiotherapy work is checked through repeated radiographic examinations.

Maintenance, Engineering and Housekeeping

These departments may not seem too important to you, at first thought, but think about them in the following terms. What is the first factor that a person notices upon walking into the hospital? You're right—how clean it is! Germs thrive in dirt—on floors, walls and furniture. The housekeeping service will cooperate with the radiology department in keeping it clean at all times. You must remember that many patients with many and varied infections come into these rooms and are radiographed on the same tables. Fresh linen is used for each patient and regularly throughout the day the tables should be wiped with an antiseptic. If a known infectious case is radiographed, all equipment and floors are thoroughly cleansed before any other patient is brought in. Windows and walls are washed at regular intervals. As a student, you should report any cleaning that needs to be done; develop good habits of cleanliness in technique and handling of patients.

We can realistically admit that the radiology department is one of the most cross-contamination prone departments in the hospital. In many departments the in-patients and the out-patients are radiographed in the same rooms at different times of the day. An out-patient could harbor some unknown infection and contaminate the equipment or room so that other patients following could pick up the infection and start a small scale epidemic. In dealing with sick people you cannot help but be aware that proper techniques in the handling of possible infectious cases are an absolute must. There is no such thing as being overly cautious when the possibility of cross-contamination exists.

The maintenance and engineering departments play an important part in the needs of the department of radiology. Our department contains some of the most complicated and expensive electronic equipment in the hospital and the number and complexity of these machines increases as time goes on. The personnel of these departments will frequently be working in the radiology department adjusting electronic equipment, heating and air-conditioning facilities, lighting fixtures and remodeling and painting in keeping with the growing needs within the department.

Laundry Service

This department takes care of the laundering of all the linen used within the entire hospital. The washing compounds must be such that all infectious germs are destroyed, because clean linen, when distributed, will be returned to the same floors but never to the same patient. All linen must be safe to use on any patient anywhere. Poor laundering techniques could cause cross-infection of all of the hospital patients. In the radiology department and in handling patients with innumerable ailments, it is imperative that linen be changed for each patient. This rule must be adhered to.

As students of radiologic technology, you must become familiar with the whole institution and the functions of each individual department. Do not wait for someone to "spoon-feed" you with information; ask about it and learn from others. Everything you learn is for your personal benefit, for the patient, and for your department. Being familiar with your institution is one of your first big responsibilities.

CHAPTER V

PERSONAL RELATIONSHIPS

Now that we have familiarized ourselves with the fundamentals of the hospital as an institution, let us return to your center of learning, the radiology department. We need to be concerned with your relationship to the other personnel with whom you have to work. You will be in contact with these individuals for hours, day after day, for two whole years. You will study and learn here; this will be possible only if your relationship with others is one of harmony and cooperation. Inasmuch as we have discussed some of these individuals in Chapter III, let us now elaborate on points relative to personal relationships.

Classmates

The size of your training school will determine the number of classmates that you have. Regardless of the number, this class will be different in attitudes and ideals from any of which you have yet been a part. You cannot harbor petty, childish attitudes toward any of your classmates as this is an indication of immaturity and would definitely hinder you in your professional work. You will all be working together, so do not look down on anyone. Perhaps you are not so exceptional, yourself, and there are people who must tolerate you. One of the secrets to success in any project is team work. Whenever there is any discontentment or disharmony, the goal cannot be reached successfully. Your classmates will be of both sexes, but at your age you should be able to work together harmoniously.

When you start your training, you may be known as freshmen or probationers; six-month students are juniors, while second year students are seniors. The junior students have just become accepted as trained, responsible student technologists. They have successfully completed the difficult preliminary adjustment, which means they show potential qualities as radiologic technologists. They may seem to ignore your class, but this is because they have ample work of their own to do. You should observe these students and their conduct. They have completed the initial phase of studies and training that you are now facing, so perhaps you could pick up a few pointers on manner of speech, conduct and professional attitudes. The juniors realize that you feel lost and uncertain and can understand your feelings. They have no right nor do they have sufficient knowledge to be capable of correcting you, but they do have some experience. Do not irritate these people by not showing them their measure of respect. Remember your place in the department, and maintain it for your own good.

The senior students are in their final year, striving to gain more knowledge, more experience and polish in their work. They are working toward graduation, the National Registry Examination and future employment in an institution of their choice. By this time they have perhaps decided to further their training and specialize either in isotope or radiotherapy technology. At the present time their primary goal is to become top-notch technologists and a credit to their profession. Many times the seniors may offer suggestions to you in your work and with your procedures. This should be for your own benefit and you have a great deal to learn from them. You should show your respect for these individuals. Any time that they devote to helping you is a contribution of their own time and interest.

The Registered Technologist

The registered technologist (referred to as the R.T.) will supervise your work at all times. He is an essential person in your training program as you cannot afford to learn by trial and error. As you learn, you will be working with actual patients; your work must be correct; patients are not used for experimentation. The supervising technologist will discuss with your instructor or chief technologist the progress that you are making in your technical or practical application. Together they will make decisions designed to aid you in improving your work. Observe his methods of conduct in dealing with the patients and someday you, too, will be capable of such professional manners.

When you have gotten to know your R.T.'s better, do not begin to take them for granted and place them at your own level. Perhaps you have established an amiable, compatible working relationship with some of the R.T.'s but this does not change your respective professional relationship. In your two short years of training you must understand that all you derive is for your own good and for the benefit of providing you with a solid background of training. The R.T.'s must expend a great deal of time and patience on your behalf and, in turn, they expect earnest, hard-working, determined students who intend to master their profession.

Invariably, there comes a time when you may learn to like certain individuals more than others. This may be due to personality types or the way that they treat you. Do not develop this attitude and deliberately try to use the friendship of any particular R. T. to gain favors. This will create a dislike for you by your colleagues, other students, and R.T.'s. This is a situation that no department can tolerate; you must treat all of the R.T.'s with equal respect. They should not and must not have favorites among the students.

In regard to personal or social relationships with the R.T.'s, it is difficult to make any fixed ground rules. From many years of experience it has been determined that there should be limitations established to preserve the professional atmosphere in the radiology department. Social contact between students and R.T.'s should be limited to the professional society social and educational functions. The private lives of the R.T.'s should not enter into the private lives of the students. The mingling of these two groups will reduce the R.T. to the same professional level as the student and carry over into the inter-relationship at work. Naturally, it could be expected that many of you will disagree on this; but, to insure the stability of the professional dignity and discipline of any department, there must be a clear distinction between students and the professional personnel.

Instructors

Your instructors undoubtedly spend many hours outside of the working day preparing assignments, lectures, correcting examinations and mapping out your training from day to day. They will try to help each of you with your own particular difficulties. They are responsible for your conduct in the department and in the presence of the patients. Many times you will think that they are strict to the point of being unreasonable, but it will not take you long to realize the absolute necessity for proper conduct at all times. It is imperative that any students who speak disrespectfully or in any way challenge the authority of any of their supervisors, the instructors, or others, should be dismissed immediately.

At the onset of your training program, the instructors will recommend certain guidelines in the number of hours that you should study per day and the methods in which to approach your assignments. In all of the years of teaching and supervising, it never ceases to amaze the author that students most always take these recommendations lightly. When their instructors state that they should study "x" number of hours per day, it seems that eight out of ten will cut that study time to about half of what was recommended. At examination time or the end of the probationary period when the time of reckoning comes and "the walls start closing in," suddenly the light dawns and the "cramming sessions" begin. In a program where practical application counts as much as theoretical knowledge, cramming will not work as it may have in high school or college. Therefore, it is recommended that you follow the study habits suggested by your instructors relative to any particular program.

Educators estimate that the human mind will forget approximately 40 per cent of the material learned. Therefore, if you only learn one-half of what you need to know and forget 40 per cent of that, you will have accomplished very little towards mastering the subject. The toughest job of any instructor is to relate this massive amount of subject material to you in a manner which you may easily assimilate. The responsibility for mastering it is yours and will come only as a result of concentrated, determined study.

Chief Technologist

The chief technologist is responsible for the productivity of his department and the conduct of his staff. This is one reason we can put emphasis on the adjective "chief." He or she will make all of the rules and regulations to be followed, and you will be expected to fall in line. Disciplinary measures and counseling will be directed by the chief technologist. Rules and regulations were determined to fulfill a specific need and you are in no position to question them. The goal of the department is to provide service to the patient by using the most effective principles and procedures.

The chief technologist will delegate duties and responsibilities to the R.T.'s and instructors, who will, in turn, delegate responsibilities to the students as a part of furthering their training. In order for the department to function properly, each individual must carry out his assignments to the best of his ability.

Associate Radiologists

Your association with the radiologists will be during special procedures and classes that they may conduct. Since radiologists are specialists, they will demand and expect that "little extra" from their staff and students. When you work with them, they will expect you to know the examination procedures thoroughly and to work efficiently. Take advantage of the efforts of these individuals to instruct you and ask intelligent questions if you do not understand a specific problem. Once it is explained to you, learn it and master it!

Chief Radiologist

The chief radiologist has a tremendous responsibility in directing the department in its service to the physicians and their patients, and to the institution as a whole. In larger centers he may be responsible for the training of resident radiologists. Everyone in the department is subject to the chief radiologist, and he is worthy of a great deal of respect in his capacity. Your contact with this individual will be minimal as he will deal with all problems relative to your training program through the school director or the chief technologist.

Attending Physician

The success of any radiology department depends upon the satisfaction of the attending physicians with the service that the department provides. Many departments depend upon cases referred to them. Undoubtedly, if service is unsatisfactory, the patients will be sent to other hospital or clinic radiology departments. This fact may not concern you too much at the present time; however, the success of your training depends upon the number and variety of examinations that you do. These determine the extent of your experience and the number and variety of examinations which you are capable of doing.

Physicians are busy individuals; their time is valuable. Usually they have numerous patients to see in the hospital, many calls to make and their office patients to see as well. Very few physicians consider their own comfort and convenience; emergencies do not arise at convenient hours. The patients are the most important individuals and their health problems are the purpose for the very existence of the medical profession. To the physician, the patients always come first and they expect the same devotion from anyone assisting them. The assistants may be nurses, laboratory technicians or radiologic technologists; the time may be day or night, but the patient's life depends upon your combined efforts. Be equally as dedicated.

The relationship of the radiologic technologist to the attending physicians should be: (1) Prompt service—in doing examinations, in making appointments, in securing radiograms in the department and in giving reports; (2) Professional conduct—undue familiarity breeds contempt. Although the physician may be a daily visitor and very friendly, be prompt, courteous and respectful; (3) Courtesy—Even if the physician is impatient or unreasonable; (4) Cooperation—in doing all examinations as requested by the physician, no matter what time of day or night. Emergencies will always be a part of our work.

At first you will not know the physicians but it is your responsibility to learn who they are, the special service they perform, and their particular requests of your department. Do not express any preferences of one physician to another. It is only natural that we would gravitate toward the friendly, courteous ones rather than those who are generally strict and demanding. If you are going to develop a professional attitude, you must realize that you need to develop a very wide latitude of acceptance towards people and their individual differences. It is doubtful that we could ever change any of them, so we must accept them as we find them.

Relative to courtesy and respect, there will be times that you will find yourself at the mercy of an irate physician. Perhaps the existing problem is not your fault; however, do not engage in any verbal disagreement with him. As a student, you may be quite sure that you will find yourself on the losing end. Whether right or wrong, you will have broken an ethical rule of conduct expected of you. Report the incident to your chief technologist, and he will solve the situation through the proper channels of authority.

Should you know a physician personally through family, church or other social contacts, do not try to carry this relationship over into your work. Regardless of how well you know this individual, in the hospital, as a physician, he assumes a position of authority and professional respect into which a personal relationship or familiarity is not acceptable.

Departmental Supervisors

The department supervisors are busy, responsible individuals whether they are nurses, laboratory technicians, therapists or non-professional personnel. In the course of working with patients, you will come in contact with all of these personnel. You will need to remember that these people will all have different personalities and mannerisms. Some of them you will find pleasant and easy to get along with; others will appear to ignore you as a student. No matter how you may try to communicate with them, they are not likely to change, so accept them as they are.

When you come onto a nursing service floor, remember that you may be a stranger to the floor personnel. Report to the nurse-in-charge before taking a patient or moving any equipment on the floor and state your purpose for being there. If you need help in moving a patient, the floor personnel will help you. The same procedure should be repeated when returning the patient. At times there will be special orders for the patient from the radiology department, and it is your responsibility to relate these orders directly to the charge nurse.

Your conduct and manners when you are away from the radiology department are very important, for they not only represent you, as a person, but the department as well. Your conduct may be interpreted as the type of training you are receiving, so it is important to maintain professional standards. Even though you may observe other professional people whose conduct is not so commendable, do not sink to their level of action. Hope that you may rise a little and elevate them with you by exercising self-restraint and dignity. There invariably comes a time when some department supervisor will attempt to make some recommendation or criticisms of you as a student. Although he or she may not have the authority to do so, do not at any time engage in verbal disagreement with this individual. Listen to the comments, then return to the department and report the incident to your chief technologist. He or she will then settle the problem as deemed appropriate. You are not in any position to engage in verbal disagreements or you will need to be disciplined for unprofessional conduct.

Hospital Employees: Professional and Nonprofessional

One condition that must be controlled is "over-friendliness" with other hospital personnel. If the relationship is of a social nature and is confined to off-duty hours outside of the hospital then there would be no particular problems involved. However, if your friends come to visit you in the department, or vice versa, then this procedure will need to be terminated immediately. Your time on professional duty should be devoted wholly to the purpose of your training. You would be wasting time that should be spent on studies, practice and concentrating on your training. You would be interrupting others in their work; no hospital department is a social center. You will have off-duty hours to spend in leisure activities and visiting your friends. It is important that you maintain your professional life and your social life as separate entities.

Religious Affiliation

Points relative to relationship with members of religious orders have been discussed in Chapter III. Here are further comments relative to the religious affiliation of the institution as a whole.

Before you enter training in any hospital, you should first investigate its particular Code of Ethics. Investigate the possibilities of conflict with your own personal beliefs in particular procedures of which you may find yourself a part. Certain procedures which are acceptable in government or privately owned hospitals are not acceptable in religiously affiliated hospitals. These will also vary from one religion to another. Consult with the school director or chief technologist and follow his recommendations and your own convictions.

The religious individuals you encounter, whether Minister, Rabbi, Priest, or Nun, should pose no problem to you as an individual. Here it should be emphasized that no matter what your own religious affiliation may be, respect the rights of others to make the same choice. Do not at any time criticize other religions or try to impose your own religion on others.

Keep in mind that no matter what the religious affiliation of any hospital may be, it exists for a single purpose—service to the sick. This service to the sick is offered to individuals no matter what their station in life may be, regardless of their religious beliefs, regardless of their wealth or lack of it. This service is provided for those in need, because *every one of us* is subject to the human frailties at some time in our lives. Disease and injury have no preference as to race, religion or creed, wealth or station in life.

CHAPTER VI

PERSONAL APPEARANCE, ATTITUDES AND HYGIENE

UP to this point we have discussed all of the people with whom you will come in contact, the patients, personnel and physicians. Let us now concentrate on you as individuals and the impressions you give to others. Perhaps you do not realize how closely you will be observed; how important it is that the impression you create is favorable. One of the factors that we must consider is personal hygiene; you must be neat, clean and tidy. Your personal appearance and hygiene must never be in question when working in such close proximity with patients and other personnel.

Personal Cleanliness

Since you were a young child, at home and at school you have been taught the basic fundamentals of personal hygiene. Let us review these fundamentals and their necessity.

Body odor results from the accumulation of perspiration and body wastes on the skin. These cannot be camouflaged by perfumes or deodorants but must be washed off. Bathing or showering is a daily must, plus the use of an effective body deodorant to protect you during the day's activities. This necessity varies from one person to another. In our type of work you come in very close contact with the patient. Perhaps you will lean over a patient while positioning him on the table. Can you imagine his discomfort at being overcome by unpleasant body odor? Female technologists should also pay particular attention to personal hygiene during their menstrual periods.

If possible, technologists should be required to wear street clothes to and from the hospital, and change at the hospital. One of the reasons for this is that in transit you may come in contact with the general public on busses and commuters. If you wear your duty uniform, there is a remote possibility that you may be carrying an infectious germ on your clothing from some patient on whom you did radiography. Consequently, through clothing contact with the general public, you might spread some of these germs to the general public. After work, the soiled uniform should be removed and sent to the laundry; showering is recommended. During the day you may have picked up any number of infectious germs on your body. Not only is this hazardous to you, but, at the same time, you may carry them home to your family. A point of equal consideration is that you may pick up germs on your clean uniform on the way to work and spread them to your patients.

Shoes are another great offender in the carrying of germs from one area to another. Duty shoes should be worn in the hospital only.

Hair is a collector of germs but for practical purposes it isn't possible to wash one's hair daily. It should, however, be washed frequently so that it will always be neat and clean.

One factor we may not take seriously enough is the problem of halitosis or bad breath. Teeth should be brushed after each meal for practical purposes, but no less than twice a day. If you have dental caries, this should be taken care of by your dentist. Many people may unconsciously have bad breath from eating a certain kind of food or if they have a stomach disorder. You should be particularly conscious of this factor also. There are few more distasteful situations than being confronted with someone's foul breath even when feeling well, much less when ill as a patient. The same situation applies to working in close contact with your colleagues. Each technologist has a personal obligation to be neat, clean, and pleasant to be near. Onions, garlic, and liquor are common offenders. Alcohol odor will often remain from the evening before and is very offensive. This, in itself, is bad enough; but the impression the patients may form is even worse. They will all object to it and may question your capabilities, feeling that perhaps you are suffering a "hang-over." Perhaps the patients' religion prohibits drinking; if so, they will have no confidence in you. Also, they may fear you do this frequently and cannot be trusted to keep personal facts about them in confidence. Do not feel that this is infringing on your private life, for most of us enjoy social gatherings and a drink. Reserve your celebrating for weekends or evenings *before* a day off.

Modern chemistry has made mouthwashes available to everyone. It is most difficult to turn on your television set and not be confronted with advertising on the problem of halitosis. Even though we may hold very little value in television advertising, this is one product we cannot afford to overlook. Whenever we are in contact with many people, there is nothing more offensive to other individuals than being subjected to halitosis because of neglect and lack of consideration. Proper precautions should be taken, in consideration for everyone around us.

Hair Styles and Hair Cuts

We should not overlook the problem of the newest fads—haircuts for men, styles for girls, and the patients' attitudes toward them.

The men should restrict themselves to brush cuts or neatly combed conservative styles. The long-haired, Beatle-type, protestors' hair styles are not acceptable in mature, professional circles. You should be cleanly shaven each morning and after-shave lotion used in moderation. Hair cremes should not be heavily scented as this can be very repulsive to an ill patient. Beards are not acceptable, but a small, neatly trimmed mustache could be tolerated. Whether you would be allowed to come into training with a mustache would depend upon school policy and your school director. If you are in the process of attempting to grow a mustache, reconsider it; a seedy, half-grown mustache does not present a professional appearance. We are working with the public and the patients' opinions and acceptance of you affects not only you as an individual but the profession, the department and the institution. The rebellious attitudes of high school and college students should not be reflected in an institution such as a hospital. You must be considered as a mature adult although your chronological age is not considered as such. A reminder to the men about body deodorants—the use of a deodorant is not a sign of femininity; it is just plain common sense.

The subject of women's hairstyles would fill a book in itself, so we will limit the discussion to the most practical hair styles to wear while on duty. The new and modern styles are very attractive in their proper place and at the proper time. No patient who is ill and worried about what disease he may have is going to feel too secure being radiographed by some technologist that is all decked out as though she were attending a movie premiere. He would be likely to question the point as to where her main interests lie. The patient will feel more secure in the hands of a neat, simply coiffured, professional person.

Exceptionally long hair is not acceptable for practical purposes. Losing hair on films or dragging it over a patient while positioning him is not acceptable. In the operating rooms where there are sterile fields, hair must be completely covered. If you have long hair, unless you can wear it in a neat, controlled practical hairdo, you should make a change. Changing the color of your hair from one week to the next may create varied opinions of you as to your maturity and stability, not only by the patients but by other personnel. It could be interpreted simply as a means to gain attention. You would no doubt get the attention you wanted, but the effects would not be to your advantage. Your natural color of hair undoubtedly suits your particular complexion best.

The wearing of wigs is becoming increasingly popular, and their authenticity and attractiveness is becoming increasingly more deceptive. Authentic wigs are acceptable; however, cheap imitation wigs are decidely unprofessional. If at some particular time you feel that you must wear a wig, be certain that it is firmly in place. It could fall off, should you lean over a patient and accidentally brush your wig against a tube stand. This would indeed be disturbing for the patient and embarrassing for you and the department.

Many school uniforms include professional caps for female technologists. If a cap is part of your complete uniform, you must have a conservative hairdo on which your cap can be worn properly. In any case, hair styles should be simple, neat, clean, no longer than shoulder length and kept in place with a hair net. This will keep it off sterile fields, patients, and cassettes. Hair could be lost during the preparation of a barium drink for fluoroscopic examinations. Should a patient discover a hair in his barium drink, in the middle of swallowing it, it could be decidedly unpleasant for the patient and embarrassing for you and the department.

Not infrequently we see individuals with dandruff problems, this can easily be controlled by medical or commercial means. Losing dandruff over the cassette can cause artifacts or could prove very dangerous if it falls onto a sterile field such as a myelogram tray.

Fingernails and Nail Polish

Another important factor in the discussion of personal hygiene is fingernails. They should be kept short, neatly trimmed and clean! Before we go further, one more statement: "absolutely *no* nail polish!" It is impractical and certainly lowers your professional appearance. Secondly, it chips and peels off into cassettes, causing film artifacts. Most doctors have displayed the attitude that it cheapens the apperance and lowers the professional atmosphere. In society, it is an accepted decorative cosmetic; but in a hospital, it should be banned entirely. Many girls like to wear long fingernails for appearance reasons, but in our profession they can only be a hindrance. In positioning a patient, one is required to locate various prominent processes and depressions in order to center the x-ray tube and cassette. With long fingernails you can hurt the patient when you press with your fingers to locate the landmarks, or you may accidentally scratch or bruise them. Long, dirty fingernails are unsightly and are collectors of germs. If you have long nails you will scratch and damage screens when loading and unloading cassettes. If you still do conventional tank developing, solutions collect under nails, staining them, and making them look discolored. Drops of solution from under long fingernails may stain the intensifying screens. Hands are germ carriers so they should be washed after handling each patient in order to prevent the spread of infections from one patient to another.

Cosmetics

Cosmetics are quite a controversial subject. We deal with many patients of all ages and religious affiliations. Many religions object vigorously to the use of any cosmetics and would object to personnel using them in excess. Heavy perfumes should definitely not be used; a faint cologne could be permissible. Strong perfume might be nauseating to an already ill patient. Lipstick should be used in moderation and in modest color shades. Eye shadow is definitely not proper for professional hospital personnel. Face powder, if you "must" use it, should be used lightly. Certainly you want to look feminine, but natural beauty is far more pleasing than a painted face. There is now an intriguing variety of eye and face makeup, the application of which is an occupation in itself. The wearing of these is acceptable at the right time and place, but not in a professional department. Heavy makeup decidedly cheapens the appearance of a professional individual.

Chewing Gum

Few things look as uncouth and unprofessional as an individual chewing gum while on duty. Not only does this hamper your manner of speech and distort your facial expressions, but it also demonstrates a form of irresponsibility and immaturity. The snapping of gum or the natural noises of chewing can be most distracting to the patient and definitely does not promote a good impression of the profession and the department. If you chew to clean your teeth, brush them instead; if you chew to sweeten your breath, use a mouthwash. Breath lozenges may be used inconspicuously.

Jewelry

Except for a wedding band and wrist watch, absolutely no jewelry should be worn while in uniform. Pendants have a habit of coming out of the uniform and dangling over the patient; large gaudy rings may scratch the patient; earrings are not professional in appearance.

Uniforms

Uniforms should always be neat and clean—a fresh one daily. Keep a spare available in case of accidents, as a stained or dirty uniform is neither sanitary nor professional. Male technologists should wear white trousers, jacket, shoes and socks. All should be clean and the uniform neatly pressed. Uniforms should be of a heavier cotton for both males and females. Nylon or synthetic materials in a uniform create an electrical static problem in the darkroom.

The female student technologist's uniform is a more complicated problem. The uniform should be of modest length, covering the kneecap. A short uniform is not feasible in view of the number of times a day that one must bend over. Abbreviated uniforms do not look very professional even if they are in keeping with the latest fashion. The most professional type of uniform is the bib front and back with skirt over a full length smock. This uniform may not do much for your figure, but, after all, this is not the purpose for your being in the department. Many of the latest uniforms cling to the nurse or technologist as if they were indeed a part of them. Even with the advent of the mini skirts and emphasis on the female figure, on the whole, patients are not impressed with these features of a technologist.

Uniforms should be large enough to work in comfortably, and heavier cotton uniforms prevent a common subject of hospital humor. Undergarments may be attractive when displayed on a mannequin but not as visualized through a uniform. While we are on the subject of undergarments, they should preferably be of cotton to avoid the static problem. Foundation garments should be of the supportive type and comfortable enough to allow one to move about unhampered. White clinical shoes and white nylons are a must; keep a spare pair of nylons available in case of runs as these are very unsightly. Shoes should be cleaned and polished daily.

Briefly, we have covered a few basic factors with regard to the personal cleanliness of body and dress. Patients and doctors much prefer neat, clean, professional, efficient, mature individuals in hospital work. We are presently living in a society where everyone would like to be a nonconformist and loves attention. As a nonconformist in hospital work you may get some attention, but, at the same time, you will get out of the hospital and profession. What may be glamorous and acceptable in television medical shows is not accepted in true life.

CHAPTER VII

CONDUCT RELATIVE TO CONVERSATION
WITHIN THE DEPARTMENT

EVERY student differs in personality traits; the way that he expresses himself in the quality and tone of his voice. The floor plan of the radiology department will vary from one institution to another. It may be so constructed that patients in the dressing room or adjacent rooms may be able to hear parts of conversations that are carried on between technologists, between technologists and radiologists, between technologists and physicians or between technologists and other patients.

Generally, each patient is a worried individual. It is human nature to be curious, to seek information about themselves and the results of the examinations; therefore, they have a tendency to be much more sensitive to hearing conversations. Patients sitting in the dressing rooms, either pre- or post-examination, may appear to be browsing through a book or just sitting there. However, their attention is focused on their surroundings, the voices and conversations they hear.

Patients have been known to hear snatches of conversations that were absolutely irrelevant to them, but they have immediately applied them to themselves and their conditions. In some instances, the presumed diagnosis has been quite serious, and many problems have resulted. Let me cite some classical examples of particular situations that have and/or can occur.

A patient, who had several radiograms taken, was waiting in a dressing room until the technologist, who took the radiograms, had the opportunity to view them and determine whether they were acceptable. In the meantime, the physician came by to view the radiograms taken earlier of another patient. The proximity of the viewing lights and the dressing rooms was such that the patient sitting in the dressing room could hear parts of the conversation between the physician and the technologist. As the technologist was setting up the radiograms for the physician, the physician commented about the serious condition of the patient and that he had not realized the disease was so advanced. Unfortunately, the patient in the dressing room recognized the voice of her physician and assumed that he was talking about her radiograms. The results were that the patient became extremely upset upon hearing the conversation. This patient was so emotionally disturbed that it took some time, through conversation with the physician, the radiologist and other hospital personnel, to be reassured. She had to be shown her radiograms and those of the other patient in question to set the matter straight and alleviate all of her doubts and mistrust.

Another example situation occurs when technologists may be viewing radiograms and discussing them from a technical standpoint. The supervising technologist may comment on the student's radiogram and state that it is a terrible radiogram. The patient, having heard that particular comment, would assume that these are her radiograms and conclude that they were terrible from the medical angle of an advanced disease.

Technologists should also refrain from discussing their private lives while on duty, particularly within hearing range of any patients. Discussing a "date" of the previous evening is hardly professional conversation material. The patient may form some pretty low opinions of the individuals in the department and their irresponsible actions and conversation while on duty.

There are numerous other examples that may be cited but it all boils down to one particular point—that walls have ears, that sound carries within the institution and what you say may be misinterpreted with serious results. It is imperative that you consider every remark, comment, or criticism you make, particularly if the patient is within hearing distance. The patients may relate these statements to themselves, to their own conditions and, consequently, the results may be very difficult with which to cope.

Loud giggling, cute expressions, etc., are definitely not acceptable within the department or institution. All conversations should be in a soft voice which does not carry so the individuals in the next room hear you. Professional personnel must be trained to walk quietly, to talk quietly, and conduct themselves gracefully.

CHAPTER VIII

MORAL OBLIGATIONS AND BEHAVIOR OF STUDENT RADIOLOGIC TECHNOLOGISTS

As a new student entering this profession, one of your most important outward responsibilities is in the way you conduct yourself. Your first demonstration of conduct is in your manner of speech. Your voice should be well modulated with distinct diction and pronunciation and should be pleasant to all who hear you. The use of slang expressions in your professional, medical work within the hospital is not desirable. Although slang is being accepted into the modern everyday vocabulary, it does create an impression that those who use it are irresponsible, unrestricted and lazy. In each passing generation, the older people seem to think that the young people are very irresponsible and live from day to day. Your use of language that is not appropriate in medical surroundings may carry over this feeling to the patient who may or may not be right about the young and modern youth.

Do not try to impress the other students, technologists or physicians by using any superlatives or descriptive terms the meaning of which you may not know. At the same time, use proper, formal English that will relate the exact meaning you wish to convey. When you are in a discussion with another individual, regardless of who he or she may be, it is extremely rude to interrupt this individual in the midst of a statement. Try to develop a habit of answering people after they have completed their statement. This may sound like a class in basic manners in kindergarten, but it is astounding the number of adults who do display very poor manners in this respect.

In schools of radiologic technology we are dealing with youth in the majority of cases, and usually students of both sexes. Giggling or loud outbursts of laughter, typical of this age group, should not be displayed either in the department or any place within the hospital at any time. Sound travels through walls and many people will hear you, particularly the patients. These loud outbursts of gaiety demonstrate a sense of irresponsibility as well as creating a doubt as to the sincerity of the people that work within the hospital. We must try to impress upon the public that the workers in a hospital are sincere and earnest in their endeavor to do their work to the best of their ability, because they are doing serious meaningful work.

Since within a group of people each individual personality will be different, you must realize that you will have to adapt yourselves to certain standards that are required within the institution and within our profession. The manner in which you express yourself verbally is extremely important, particularly in your manner of answering people. Answer everyone in a pleasant, sincere tone. Your tone and mannerisms should be consistent with an appreciation of the situation you are in at that time. Abrupt answers may represent annoyance, disrespect for authority or an "I couldn't care less" attitude. Therefore, your answers must be pleasant, sincere, and must express the feeling that it is a willing answer.

The fact that your voice represents you in every stage of your work and your general feelings at that specific point, it is probably one of the most important factors, as it expresses *you* as you really are. Your manner of speech, your voice and your control of it are one of the strongest tools that represent your development and you as an individual.

Behavior

Your behavior in your training school, as well as after you have graduated, represents not only you but your profession, your department and your institution. Perhaps there is the opinion held by many today that it is acceptable to "goof off," as long as you are not caught. Remember that in the medical professions, you may get away with something that is not in keeping with the behavior or conduct required, but someone else will suffer.

Being realistic is a difficult thing to face in our daily lives. Politicians, business men, and others, may cheat and take advantage of other people to make a personal profit. Individuals in our line of work—radiologic technology—must remember that if we take advantage of anyone we are taking advantage of the individual who is seeking our help: the patient. The most outstanding quality which you must understand and use every day of your life is that of being truthful. Truth and honesty are, without a doubt, absolute personality requirements. Should we cheat in any way, no matter how minute, we cannot achieve the goal of being truly professional and devoted to the services of mankind. Trying to make little excuses to cover up your forgetfulness or misuse of supplies is one of the first temptations. It happens and certainly you will also encounter many similar incidents where students will try to get away with covering up their errors. Many times students conceal their technically erroneous films from their instructors or the chief technologist, hoping to avoid disciplinary action.

Being realistic is difficult to face, but in every sense of the word, what you are doing by covering up your errors, by being deceptive, is being untrue to yourself, your school and the profession. Did you really get away with anything, and for how long? How long will it be before you repeat the same deception which sooner or later will catch up with you? Again, what have you really done? You have lowered yourself; you have lost some self-respect and personal pride in training yourself to be a truly professional technologist.

CHAPTER IX

YOUR FIRST DUTY WITH THE PATIENT

YOUR first contact with the patients will possibly be to bring them from their floor to the radiology department. In many institutions this will be your first assignment after being taught the principles of patient lifting and moving. Your attitudes, manner and conduct with the patients at this time will either put them at ease and make them feel secure or make them question the capabilities of the personnel of the radiology department.

My purpose in discussing this is to make you realize just how much responsibility there is in doing a relatively simple task. When you enter the patient's room, greet him according to the time of day and inform him of your name and the department you represent. Ask the patient his name and see if it corresponds exactly with the name on the requisition. Establish the following information: the patient's full name, age, and his doctor's name. After he has answered your questions and the information corresponds, confirm it also by checking the name bracelet.

You should never ask a patient, "Are you Mr. Jones?" The patient may be drowsy from sleep or under light sedation and would nod his head in agreement, thinking that you had said "Mr. James." This type of error should not occur, but it can and has happened to technologists. Just think for a moment what could happen. The following extreme example can be visualized in varying degrees of severity.

Mr. James is taken to the radiology department for the type of radiologic examination as specified on the requisition. If the information is not confirmed in the radiology department (which could happen on a busy day, if someone else is also careless), Mr. James' radiograms would be labeled with Mr. Jones' name. The radiologist would not be aware of the error and would make the diagnosis on the radiograms under the name of Mr. Jones. Suppose that Mr. James (who was radiographed) had a lesion requiring surgical removal and surgery is done on Mr. Jones instead. Do you see the importance of establishing the identity of a patient beyond any doubt? This is why you must be constantly alert and conscious of the possibility of error; the patient is relying upon your knowledge. Double check yourself if there is even the slightest doubt.

As you enter the patient's room, you must realize that your facial expression, the tone of your voice and your general attitude will affect the attitude of the patient. If you enter the room in a professional manner, not overly cheerful but pleasant, his rather questionable day may be lightened and brightened by your general outlook. You may be responsible for making his day brighter by contributing to a cheerful, pleasant atmosphere. Do not enter the room asking questions in a brusque, precise manner, sounding like a broken record and with about as much feeling. This may put the patient in a "braking attitude." Not only will he be tempted to be uncooperative, but he may become uneasy and impatient with you. Your initial exchange of words with a patient may be the determining factor between a successful examination with the patient being cheerful and cooperative or the exact opposite.

When coming for a patient, always check first with the charge nurse on the floor; state your name, your department, the name of the patient you have come for and the type of examination he is to have. In smaller hospitals the staff may know you, but in very large institutions identity is important and courtesy promotes good interdepartmental relationship. Patients have been known to walk out of hospitals, and if you do not report taking a patient from the floor, you could create quite a commotion and search. The nurse may also have further information that you need concerning the patient. When all this is completed, you may take your patient to the radiology department.

After completion of the scheduled examination, you may be requested to return the patient to his bed. Be absolutely certain that the patient is taken to the correct room and bed, and report again to the nurse. At this time relay any orders from the radiology department; e.g., the patient may eat; the patient may not eat; or certain medications need to be given as prescribed by the radiologist. These orders are important to the success or failure of the examination itself and must be relayed without delay. When you return the patient to his room, ask if there is anything that you can do in the way of assuring his comfort (getting him a drink of water, a magazine, adjusting the bed, etc.). Thank your patient politely for his cooperation in assisting in having the radiography done. It is important that you leave the patient with as pleasant a memory of the radiology department as possible to insure future cooperation if further radiography needs to be done on him.

Perhaps now you understand more clearly the importance of making the visit of each patient to the department of radiology pleasant and reassuring in the service that you have provided, and the importance of doing a seemingly simple task well. There are many tragic errors that could result from the actions of a careless, irresponsible person.

CHAPTER X

RELATIONSHIP AND ATTITUDES
TO THE PATIENT

Special Consideration for the Patient

LET us now come to the main objective of this book—how to overcome situations arising from contact with many and varied patients. What will be your relationship with the patient? How do you look at these various problems? How will you go about solving them?

At present, perhaps all patients seem more or less the same to you. Perhaps they may differ only in how ill they are. Many patients will be on the critical list, but most of them will be in for a check-up because they have some particular problem. Never are you to set yourself up as a judge of how sick they are. You will do only your best work at all times and maintain the highest quality of radiograms taken.

We should show sympathy for and understanding of the patient. We must take human beings as we find them; the irritable, unreasonable, over-exacting patients cannot be transformed and at no time should we try. Technologists will have to learn early how to size up the type of patient and adapt themselves to the personality problem involved. All patients must be treated with sympathy and understanding, never disbelief. An irritable patient may be soothed by a tactful technologist; never become irritated and show it. By being pleasant and even-tempered, you may improve the patient's manner. He may become aware of his poor behavior and apologize. No matter if you think it is due you, never convey this attitude to him. Make him feel at ease, and show your understanding of the reasons for his attitudes, such as illness, worry, or tension. Never show resentment.

On the other hand, had you retorted when the patient displayed his childish behavior, most likely he would have become more irritable and probably would have refused to let you do anything for him. You might have found yourself being reported to your superiors. In this case, we both know that although the patient was basically in the wrong, you will stand on the losing side and could very easily be dismissed from training. This is why a competent technologist must possess an even temper and an endless amount of patience and understanding. If you find it difficult to practice self-control, then you are planning on the wrong profession. You could search endlessly but never find a spot where every patient would be cheerful and pleasant. We are fortunate that most of them are reasonable, but it is by the few others that we are tested.

One of the successful approaches in establishing rapport with the patient is to demonstrate the positive approach in your desire to help him. The patient is a stranger in the hospital expecting and seeking help from his physician and everyone with whom he comes in contact. When the patient is having radiography done on him, he is looking up to you as an individual who will do your job to the best of your ability, and the resulting radiograms will demonstrate his problem to his physician. You must emanate an attitude of authority and confidence that you do possess all the knowledge necessary to obtain the best quality radiogram. You must conduct yourself in an organized manner; you must demonstrate to the patient that everything you are doing in the room is important and that you thoroughly understand everything about you. Even though you may only be in your late teens or early twenties, you must act mature and responsible to show you are qualified for the task before you. The manner in which you move about, handle the equipment and instruct the patient in helping to maintain a specific position has to demonstrate complete mastery of the procedure.

Patients have a notoriously poor memory for past examinations, so have we all. They may have had radiography done in your department only a matter of months before but just cannot remember the date. As a test, try to recall when you last saw your doctor or dentist, or when you had your glasses changed. It isn't all that easy, is it? So, if a patient has a difficult time recalling something, don't stand there with a look on your face that says, "how dumb can you get?" Remember, these people are ill or they would not be scheduled for radiography. They are tense, nervous, and worried. Strive to help them in approximating the year, the season, and finally even the month of their last examination. Do you perhaps see now how a little tact and consideration can be priceless virtues? Whenever you feel yourself losing these, just put yourself in the patient's place and everything will return to its proper perspective.

Your Personal Reactions and Feelings Toward the Patient

Your personal feelings toward any patient should be a desire to help them to the best of your ability. You should refrain from showing undue emotion and always remain calm, friendly, and reserved, as the situation demands. It is not meant that you be indifferent, but as a professionally trained person, you must be in command when put in the midst of tense, highly emotional situations. You will witness many of these and you may find yourself as the only calm person there. Perhaps an example would serve to explain this in a better way.

Frantic parents have rushed a small child to the emergency room. She is cyanotic and barely breathing, has a high fever and has had vomiting and diarrhea for two days. She has a seizure right on the emergency room table. No doubt, as the doctor aids the child's breathing he will also ask for a chest radiograph, but, as you stand there, film cassette in hand, the child expires. She was brought in too late! Such a beautiful, innocent child! Why did she have to die? As mortal men, who are we to ask? God is our Creator. He has put us here for a time and with a purpose. It was not meant that we should always understand why. The parents are overcome with grief and their expressions of emotion may affect you deeply, but you must practice self-control. You have done your best, and that is all you could be expected to do. This is a solemn moment—only one of many.

Perhaps another example could be of this nature. A rebellious teen-ager was critically injured in a drag race, and, from the odor on his breath, it was evident he had consumed much alcoholic beverage. Perhaps you will think, how disgusting! He has injured himself, brought grief upon his family and friends. Should you feel contempt or pity? Try not to make any judgments of this nature, for they are not yours to make. Do the requested radiography to the best of your ability with one purpose in mind—to help him as much as you can. His actions and attitudes were developed by some negative source of influence which you may never know about or understand. You will encounter many and varied situations, and you will have to adapt yourself to cope with all of them in a professional manner.

Reassurance

The patients coming for radiologic examinations may be frightened. They may be afraid of what the examinations will reveal. Perhaps they have read all the articles on the physical bodily harm that can result from excessive radiation. Sometimes they are afraid simply because they do not understand; this is a completely new experience. They don't know what to expect and must be reassured.

Do not approach the patients with a facial expression as if to say: "my, my, you poor soul, what a pitiful sickly individual you appear." Approach your patients with a smile and kind greetings and try to put them at ease. An explanation of the procedure to follow will show the patients that you know what you are doing and wish to do your best. A basic understanding of what is expected of them will enable the patients to cooperate fully so that you can obtain good quality radiograms. Just why some technologists expect to get patients to cooperate in "taking a deep breath and holding it" during a chest examination, without a word of explanation, is still the sixty-four dollar question. The fact that you do not bother to inform or explain to the patient gives him the impression that you do not care, and just want to get the examination done. Never actually develop this attitude, for you will have ruined yourself and the prestige of your department and profession.

Repeatedly you will encounter patients who deliberately refrain from helping you in trying to get a good radiogram; there may be many reasons that cause this lack of cooperation. They may be uncooperative in maintaining certain positions such as keeping the shoulders forward for a postero-anterior chest view. If they fail to maintain the exact position for either an antero-posterior or postero-anterior view, you will probably obtain an oblique view. Do not demonstrate annoyance with this type of individual; use various restraining devices in trying to do the view independently of the patient.

The patient may fail to cooperate with you because he is too ill; he doesn't want to have this examination done but his physician does, or for the price of radiographic examinations these days he feels you can do it without his help. The latter is not unusual with the current discontent of high medical costs. Whatever the situation may be, we must remain courteous and helpful to the fullest extent, regardless of what our personal opinions or feelings may be. Do not develop an attitude of indifference to this type of patient as it will tend to carry over into all of your work.

Courtesy

Each individual patient has a right to be treated with courtesy. This does not mean you must kowtow and call everybody "sir," but maintain a respectful, kindly attitude with everyone. Your attitude must be one of interest in your work and a desire to help. If a patient arrives five minutes before the end of your working day it may not be his fault. Do not express annoyance but handle the situation tactfully. If the examination can be done, then do it. The patient may not be able to come the next day for he may not be able to get time off from his job. Always keep in mind the patient's side of the story and, as a devoted professional person, try to help.

Modesty

All patients have varied degrees of modesty. Take the clothes away from any patient, give him a patient gown, and you take away something else, too; his confidence. Probably he feels like two cents. No patient should be expected to undergo a radiologic examination with anything less than a clean, long gown that covers him adequately.

After months or years in your work, you may sometimes get

a little careless in covering the patients properly. However, remember that the patients are very conscious of this. Exposure is unforgiveable and something that the patients are not likely to forget or forgive. It doesn't matter if the patients are eight years old or eighty, they are all modest. Modesty is a personal virtue and should be respected, especially if it is someone else's.

People vary along a wide margin in their manners and conduct. Some patients are so frightened at the thought of disrobing and putting on a gown that their actions are almost ridiculous. Other people are so careless and carefree that you will find yourself embarrassed. If you have ever been led to believe that women are more modest than men, this is not so.

We are taught at an early age to respect personal modesty and it is a cherished virtue if it is sincere. If you should carelessly expose any patient during an examination, you have degraded the patient in his own eyes. Can you possibly understand the embarrassment if you should meet on the street at some later date? It would be embarrassing to this type of patient to be recognized by you, inasmuch as he had been seen without clothes. Such patients will probably never come to your hospital again, and it will be because of your thoughtlessness.

In positioning dozens of patients every day, on occasion, a sheet could accidentally slip off, exposing the patient. This could happen to a patient getting on or off the table or because of a required position for examination which may be awkward. In such a situation you will tactfully cover the patient as if nothing happened and proceed in your work.

There are other patients who could not seem to care less whether they are covered at all. In such a situation, you will efficiently wrap a sheet around them to cover what the gown seems to have missed. This must be done tactfully and without reprimand; the patient must not be embarrassed for his own lack of modesty. Still other patients would not feel secure even if they were wrapped in six sheets. By facial expression or action, never make them feel childish because of their fears. We are not likely to reform them, so deal only with the immediate situation.

A situation the author finds rather puzzling is that female technologists and nurses are allowed to do procedures for male patients without being questioned. Since the days when Florence Nightingale worked with male patients, society has accepted it as fitting and proper. Female technologists should not be expected to administer enemas or catheterize male patients, young or old. Oppositely, the same should be the rule for male technologists. This situation proves very embarrassing for the patients. There will sometimes be exceptions in small outlying hospitals where it is a matter of sheer necessity. We should follow as closely as possible a rule in medical ethics applying to doctors. Ethically, no male doctor should examine a female patient unless accompanied by a nurse or vice versa for female doctors. Patients are quite resentful toward anyone who does not respect their modesty.

It is always the responsibility of the technologist to see that his or her patients are properly attired. Never leave the patients and expect them to find their way to the dressing room, waiting room, or lavatory. Take the patients to these rooms yourself for they may inadvertently enter the wrong room. Can you imagine the scene if Mr. Jones, on his way to the dressing room, would accidentally make his way into Mrs. Smith's dressing room instead? Just suppose Mrs. Smith was standing there in her "birthday suit" reaching for her gown! Mrs. Smith and Mr. Jones will both probably end up in the administrator's office with a legitimate complaint. Can you blame them? Do you suppose either of them will ever come back to your hospital again? Probably not, and, to make matters worse, they will advise their friends of the careless, thoughtless treatment they received. The story of this incident, magnified at each telling, will spread to countless people in a short time. Can you now see your responsibility to the patients and to the hospital? Each worker, professional and nonprofessional, is morally obligated to uphold and protect the reputation of the institution for which he works.

You may sometimes become careless with patients of your own sex and think nothing of seeing them exposed. Just reverse the situation and imagine how you would feel as the patient. Surely you would want to be kept covered.

Occasionally, you will have patients of the opposite sex who appear deliberately careless in getting on and off the table. They may just be careless or may be mentally ill. You are not here to diagnose the mental condition of the patients. Your only alternative is to quietly and skillfully cover the patients and proceed with the examination. They can be wrapped in sheets to make skirts not likely to slip off. The patients may see from your professional attitude that they are not making an impression and will behave properly.

There are patients who are overly self-conscious about wearing a gown and sheet. If the patients are overly modest, do not make it difficult for them to preserve their own desired level of modesty. You will find this particularly true with the female patients. Even though you have asked the patient repeatedly to undress "completely" and put on a gown and sheet, she will insist on keeping on articles of clothing, particularly her bra and panties. If it is absolutely necessary to remove these undergarments for the success of this examination, kindly but firmly explain that they must be removed or they will show up on the radiogram and complicate the problem of rendering an accurate diagnosis. Do not become impatient and demand that the patient remove her garments, as you may find her refusing to continue the examination. If the patient insists on covering herself with several sheets, accept this graciously and continue with the examination as best you can. If you insisted on limiting the number of covers, you may have found the patient complaining of your lack of consideration and defiantly report to her physician that you had exposed her unnecessarily. This is always a very unpleasant situation and can create quite a problem for you and the department.

Regardless of the fact that we live in the age of mini skirts and topless bathing suits, the general public is not so brazen as a rule. In the hospital people may become either very self-conscious or the exact opposite. You must also consider the age of the patient and the possible presence of emotional disturbance. We must preserve the patient's dignity for, or in spite of themselves. There are numerous ways to handle such situations, and you will be confronted with many. You must learn to control your facial expression. You must never register surprise or make the situation worse by blushing. Try to maintain your composure by your facial expression and in the continuation of the examination.

When positioning or doing special examinations, let your attitude towards patients be impersonal but not indifferent. Familiarity is not ethically acceptable. A complaint from patients could very easily result in your dismissal from training.

Religious Affiliation

There are some basic factors which enter into our discussion on the personal relationships with our patients. One of these factors is religion. The basic purpose of our profession is to serve our fellow man in his hour of need. We must serve the sick, no matter what their religious affiliation. We are not qualified to judge the right or wrong of different religions. Never, never should we begrudge a person care or treatment because we do not personally believe in his religion. Even in our great country, where the right to worship as we wish is a personal choice, we are plagued with prejudice. Religion often becomes a political football. Our society is full of bigots, and we, as individuals, are not likely to change them. As mature, intelligent individuals we can do one thing: that is to keep our profession free from religious prejudice.

Many times in the course of conversation with patients you may find yourself asked this question, "What is your religion?" Now this may seem like a harmless question at the time but it "could" have repercussions. Perhaps that particular patient disagrees with your religion. Perhaps that patient dislikes all members of your particular religion. If this is the case, he will probably distrust you and refuse to let you do the examination. On the other hand, he may just be politely uncooperative and try to get you in trouble by complaining to the radiologist. Your best answer to the question of religion is that you do not discuss it on duty, that you feel it is the private concern of every individual. This must be done tactfully and in a friendly manner. Even if the patient is of the same religious faith as yours, religion is still a good subject to avoid. The patient may develop a strong personal attachment to you and become overly friendly.

Race

Along with religion we also encounter another problem in society, and that is the one of race. In this country there are certain areas where this is a major problem. It is not our aim here to solve the racial problem but to deal with it as far as it concerns the profession of radiologic technology. If we have been in contact with these racial differences and harbor these ideas ourselves, we may find work in a medical profession rather difficult. Remember that all men are created equal in the eyes of God. Upon graduation, it is a part of the context of our oath that we treat and serve all men equally. We should not allow problems created by society to influence our treatment of any race different from our own. All patients should be treated equally. Segregation cannot be allowed to enter any of the medical professions as it has many others. Our profession was formed for the express purpose of service to our fellow man in his illness. Perhaps we should turn to the words, "Inasmuch as ye have done it unto the least of these, My brethren, ye have done it unto Me."

Social Standings

In our profession, we are continuously in contact with people of all ages, religions, races, and, of course, social standings. Walking down the street we see the wealthy, the middle class, the average worker, those who are just plain poor and the social welfare class. There is very little or no social interrelationship between these classes. In the hospital we will come in contact with members of each of these classes. Disease and death do not play favorites; neither should we. A patient should be someone we can help because he is ill no matter whether or not he has a dollar. It is unethical to render better care to a patient just because he can afford a private room or drives the fanciest car. Everyone should be given the utmost care and all examinations should be done to the best of our ability. It might be quite a temptation to take care of Mrs. Jones, who owns half of the town, and let Mr. Smith, an alcoholic who depends upon social welfare, sit and wait. We cannot be true to ourselves or our profession if we discriminate between our patients according to their social standing.

Age

From the unborn child to the very old and infirm, sickness may affect all. As we progress in our training, we will find our most difficult patients to be the very young and the very old.

If we find ourselves cringing at the thought of doing radiography on a ninety-year-old person and dislike having to do it, remember that perhaps our grandparents will soon be that old. Has it ever occurred to you that in a few score years we will be "old" too? How would we like to have our family or ourselves treated in a similar situation? Remember that it is very difficult for children or the very old to understand and cooperate; they depend upon us. Therefore, this is one situation that requires our patience, knowledge, and skill. In everyday life these helpless patients depend upon their parents or their children. It should be a real challenge to us in our work, and doing a good job should be our satisfaction.

Meeting Former Patients in Public

Our personal relationship with the patient does not always begin and end in the hospital. We may face a situation in public that will require some quick thinking on our part. We will meet former patients walking down the street, in the department store, or at a public function. Sometimes we may even encounter former patients in the homes of friends. In such a circumstance we will have to judge whether these people wish to be remembered. If their experience in the radiology department was brief and surrounded by normal circumstaces, they may be quite pleased to be recognized and called by name. However, if there were unpleasant factors present they might just be happy that we do not remember them.

At first you may remember all of your patients for they undoubtedly will make quite an impression on you. Later in your training you will find yourself remembering only the unusual ones. Many of you and your instructors may disagree with the author. For practical purposes, the following examples may be used to explain.

Suppose you are uptown shopping and a man taps you on the shoulder. He smiles and says "hello." You soon recognize "Mr. Jones" and remember radiologic examinations that he had at the hospital. Do you greet him by name and ask him how his ailment is, or what do you do?

Early in your training you should train yourself to forget names and examinations of your patients. In time you will have done so many it will be impossible to remember them anyway.

Let us return to Mr. Jones, whom you have encountered on the street and is about to start a conversation. Your first reaction should be to ask his name and where you've met before. He might continue by telling you how you had "x-rayed" him and how well you had done. You should deny remembering these facts. He may then bring up all sorts of occurrences to try to get you to remember. Even if you do suddenly remember him, continue to deny it. This is one important reason: he may be one of the many who really do not wish to be remembered. There may have been unpleasant or embarrassing moments during his examination that he would rather you had forgotten. His one fear is that if you do remember, you may tell others about it or use him as an example. This would be an invasion on his personal privacy which you have no right to divulge. Assure your former patients of this right, and they will respect you for it.

The following example is one of the author's own experiences, and this particular incident shall never be forgotten. At approximately midnight, one Saturday, a patient was brought into the emergency room with what appeared to be a broken nose. It seems she and her husband had quarreled and he had struck her in the face, injuring her nose. The only persons, up to this time, who were aware of this incident were Mr. and Mrs. X, the doctor, the emergency room attendant, and myself. Radiograms were taken to determine the extent of injury and proper care was administered. Mr. and Mrs. X, needless to say, were quite embarrassed by the whole affair.

Some weeks later while at a private party, the guests being introduced included Mr. and Mrs. X. While shaking hands with Mrs. X, she exhibited a particular uneasiness. Although not remembered immediately, there was something familiar about her; however, this was soon dismissed from my mind and the evening progressed happily. It did occur to me that I was being watched closely by Mrs. X. Later in the evening she approached me and asked if I remembered her. Suddenly it dawned on me exactly who she was and I found myself in a very delicate situation. This individual's self-respect had to be protected, I denied ever having known her, or having met her. I assure you I was given the first degree, but explained that as a professional person I had been trained not to remember or discuss any patients outside of the hospital. I could see the look of relief on her face as she was assured I did not recall the incident and would not reveal her secret. (It might be added, she and her husband were socially prominent people.) Mrs. X appeared to enjoy the party much more during the remainder of the evening.

The world is a very small place and you meet many former patients in public. It is better not to recognize them, thus leaving their minds at ease; you cannot really cause any harm by forgetting.

Often, you may be confronted with a situation whereby you will work with former patients on public projects such as in a club fund-raising project or sponsoring a social function. If people start questioning you, you should deny remembering any cases you have done. People are often just plain "nosey" and will try to obtain information on various cases, types of cases, how they are handled, etc. These individuals will then go among their friends and relay your information, usually distorted more at each telling. They will tell how all the cases are handled and things that go on in the hospital that no one finds out about. You will see you should never discuss your department, your work or your institution with anybody outside the hospital. You may damage irreparably your professional reputation and the reputation of the profession.

Many individuals like to isolate themselves from one another. People seem to have a certain number of secrets about themselves and their families that they would rather no one know, particularly the personnel in the hospital. It is true that some of the patients come to the hospital under adverse conditions. They may be intoxicated or involved in a situation contrary to or unacceptable by social standards; consequently, they would not like their friends and neighbors to know about it. Undoubtedly, these patients would be embarrassed if recognized by personnel from the hospital at some later time. They very likely are trying hard to forget the incident that brought them to the hospital.

In summary, it may be better not to remember your patients

or recognize them in public since all you know about them should remain within the walls of the institution. Your public confrontations with the patient should not bring up the topic of your knowledge about them or whatever ailed them or how you came to know them at the hospital.

Gifts or Tips

In our society "tips" are bestowed upon individuals for services rendered. Often you will be offered a tip by a patient. Even though you have worked hard and may deserve a reward, you should not accept it. Why? A medical professional individual does not accept tips. The principle of this should be tactfully explained to the patient. You can tell the patient, if he is pleased with your work, that he may express thanks to the department head and the hospital administration. Tell him that he was an excellent patient, and you couldn't help but do efficient work with his cooperation. This will create a good relationship between the patient and the hospital, as well as the public to whom he will convey his feelings. The exception to this rule is that you may accept a gift that may be shared by the whole department, such as candy, flowers, etc. This can be considered as a token of appreciation. Be sure to return the courtesy extended with a "thank you" card.

CHAPTER XI

HOW TO DETECT THE PERSONALITY
TYPE OF YOUR PATIENT

W E have discussed some of the personality types and possible methods of working with them; let us now dwell on the subject of detecting them. It is very important that we detect the type of persons we are going to radiograph. Knowing the type of personality can eliminate a great number of misunderstandings and allow you to communicate with patients more effectively. The following are but a few of the types that will be encountered.

QUIET TYPE. As a rule these patients may be the polite, soft-spoken type of individuals. They usually appear as the bashful type who would like to start a conversation but do not have the courage. The technologist must be careful not to approach these patients in a manner too bold or businesslike. This could make the individuals nervous and cause them to fear you. When you detect this type of person, put forth some extra effort to be pleasant and courteous. Usually they will soon start to come out of their shell of reserve and you will find an intelligent, cooperative, and friendly type of person. As a rule, they are very patient and understanding; if they have to wait while the department is busy, they seldom complain. Because of this, we may sometimes overlook the quiet patients and pay more attention to the grumbling, impatient ones. For this reason, again it is stressed, treat each of your patients with equal respect. Do not take advantage of the quiet type and push them in a corner simply because they do not voice a strong opinion because of the delay. We could probably classify the quiet type as a mild form of introversion.

MOODY TYPE. One of our main problems is the "moody" type: gay one minute and pouting the next. This type is hard to handle properly because they are so unpredictable. Their moods may change from one day, one hour, or one minute to the next. If you meet them in a relatively good mood, try to carry through in the same atmosphere, for if you put them in a bad mood they will complain and usually magnify any problem that occurs. If you are pleasant when they are gay, you will usually end up with a cooperative effort in taking the radiograms. If you encounter them in an irritable mood, do not add more fuel to the fire. Be pleasant and you will find the mood is contagious and will catch. They will often become happy because of your attitude. Should they not change, no matter how much they may irritate you, do not retaliate. If your mood remains pleasant, they will soon realize their error. If you cannot change their mood, at least don't give them any reason to complain about you. Do not lower your behavior to their level; rather, maintain a pleasant, courteous professional attitude.

EXTROVERT. The extroverts may be a problem to technologists. For one thing, they are usually the loud, boisterous type and may tend to treat you as just another nobody. Do not let these individuals irritate you but proceed with your work in a quiet, professional manner. These individuals are often impressed with fast, efficient workers. Carry on a normal type of conversation if the individuals wish, and be courteous even if you feel like being otherwise. If you work with speed and efficiency, their attitudes toward you may change and they may even compliment you. Be polite and professional in accepting any compliments and proceed with your work. Should you need to repeat a radiogram because of poor technique or positioning, do not tell this to patients. Tell them it is for the confirmation of previous radiograms. Here again, never give the patients a reason to complain about you; if you succeed in this, you have beaten them at their own game.

IMPATIENT PATIENT. One of the most common problems and the hardest to bear is the "impatient patient." These individuals have no consideration for anyone or anything except themselves. They expect you to drop everything and attend them as soon as they arrive, especially if they are out-patients. They think they are kings and you are their servants. Aside from being impatient, they are rude and demanding. Neither you nor I will change them and by resisting them we will only increase the unpleasantness of the situation. When this type of individual arrives, do your best to get them done and out of the front door as soon as possible. If they are early, remind them of it and tell them you will take care of them as soon as possible. If your room is occupied because of an emergency, tell them it is occupied and ask them if they can come back later. Give yourself plenty of time so that you will be ready for them when they return. Send them to the cafeteria if their examination allows them to eat or drink, or anywhere that will make the time pass more quickly. If they remain, the only way to keep them quiet is to work quickly and efficiently. If they see that you are really quite busy, which you should be, they will be less impatient about awaiting their turn.

If these individuals are in-patients, do not bring them to the department until you are ready for them. If they must wait until the films are processed, explain the reason and approximate the time you will be taking them back to their room. Add a few extra minutes to the time you will actually need. In this way, if you are finished earlier than they expected, they will be pleased that you hurried for them.

The impatient individual cannot be changed. He will try to impress you with his own importance and that he has no time to wait; he expects to be waited upon and treated as someone of importance. As intelligent professional people, we will not try to diminish this self-importance. Do not aggravate this type of person in any way; treat all with respect.

SUSPICIOUS TYPE. The suspicious type is wary of you and watches your every move. These patients are often suspicious that you are taking too many exposures and running up the bill. They ask many questions. Explain to them that the number of radiograms does not indicate the cost, as prices are set per examination rather than the number of radiograms. Explain also that several views are needed to determine the diagnosis and are requested by the radiologist, not by yourself. They will ask you the results of the radiograms for they are suspicious of what they may have, the biggest fear being cancer. Likely they will not believe what you tell them anyway, and often will be suspicious of you as a person, perhaps you appear uncertain or carefree or display any other of numerous actions. You must conduct yourself in a sincere, courteous, professional manner and emanate confidence. If they ask you questions, answer them to the best of your ability within ethical allowances. If you do not know the answers, refer them to the chief technologist who will be glad to answer what is permissible. They could also be told to ask their personal physician. Never avoid their questions for they will only become more suspicious of you, the department, and the hospital. If they actually voice any suspicions they have, clear them up; if you cannot, then refer them to someone who can. Instill confidence in them for their own sake. Show them that people in the medical profession are devoted individuals working for the benefit of their patients. Try to make them feel that there is a purpose and a benefit in medical care and it is to their advantage.

HYPOCHONDRIAC. The hypochondriac patient is the one who *thinks* he has a disease and is suffering terribly. There are quite a number of people who imagine and fear they have one or more diseases and they actually experience the pain. Although the doctor may not be able to find anything wrong organically, the pain suffered is real. Perhaps they need and want attention and this is the only method by which they can get it. You will perhaps be able to get more cooperation from this type of patient if you can divert their minds temporarily to some other interest. Find a topic of popular interest and engage the patient's mind, meanwhile proceed with positioning of the patient and the examination. You may find they really are able to move about better than they think. Remember again that these patients are actually in pain, so handle them accordingly. Be sympathetic, but in moderation. The hypochondriac needs and wants sympathy. Remember also that you are in no position to judge, so never tell them they do not have any pain or illness. Do not be overly sympathetic or you may find this type of patient forming an attachment to you and asking you to come and visit them; therefore, keep your friendship on a professional basis. If these patients should start to insist upon you sharing your time with them, explain to them kindly that the rules and regulations do not allow students to visit socially among the patients. We must be very careful not to suspect too many of our patients to be hypochondriacs. This problem is for the doctor to solve.

It has been experienced that a patient would object to having a joint moved even before the subject was approached. If the pain in this joint came on without injury, then there is some question. There have been occasions when the joint could be bent very slowly and carefully while the patient was engaged in a sincere discussion. This is a trick and should not be used except by a well-experienced senior student or a graduate technologist after having seen it done many times. This can be a delicate situation and you may upset the patient. You must possess a great deal of tact and skill before attempting anything of this nature.

Basically, you should try to take the patient's mind off his pain and he will cooperate more fully.

Handling of Various Types of Intoxicated Patients

We will be called upon to handle patients in all conditions, which include those under the influence of alcohol or drugs. The most common will be the intoxicated patients with their many problems. These problems will be varied in respect to their actions, their conduct and their general behavior. Perhaps from the following examples of some of the more major problems and situations, you will be able to apply these suggestions to situations you, yourself, will encounter. These may guide you to make decisions on your own. Let us now discuss a few of the personality types.

YOUNG ABUSIVE TYPE. The young violent type of male patient is one of the most difficult to handle. Such people, as a rule, object to medical treatment including radiograms and will repeatedly tell you they are all right. They may be abusive and try to upset you and cause more trouble. Probably the best way to handle this situation is not to argue with them but just let them ramble on with their complaints. They may also curse everyone in sight, including you, but do not let yourself be upset by it. Upsetting you is one of their aims, so do not give them the chance. Do your work quickly and try to finish as soon as possible. If these patients should ask questions, answer them politely and precisely, but do not engage in any lengthy conversation. If the patients start to aggravate you and be abusive to you directly, tell them simply that you have been asked by their physicians to do the examinations and that you are not obliged to take any abuse from them.

Ask them politely to keep their comments to themselves. If, after hurling abuse upon you, they should realize what they have done and start to apologize, accept the apology and go about your work. If, however, the patients should become more insulting, tell them you will call in a doctor and have him handle the situation. In most instances these patients are usually brought in by the police or must be reported to the police so your greatest problem is under control when an officer is present.

The female technologists will invariably come across young intoxicated males who suddenly become Rudolph Valentino with as many arms as an octopus. If you should get very stern or insulting you may rile them up to the point where they would become abusive and try to harm you. You should ward them off tactfully, saying something like: "Why, Mr. Jones, what would your wife (or girl friend) say if she could hear you now?" Try to pay very little attention to the romantic phrases and proceed with your work as though you had not heard them. Be professional, do not smile or you may just lead them on. Do not allow them any opportunity to place a hand on you in any way. If one should, take his hand in a firm grip and put it by his side; express no opinion the first time. If he should attempt it a second time, tell him politely that such conduct is not permitted and seek help if necessary. If any intoxicated young male patients are to be undressed for the required examinations, make sure they are sufficiently covered; do not allow them an opportunity to expose themselves. The intoxicated young male patient is best calmed down by having a male attendant present in the room while he is being radiographed by a female technologist. The presence of the male will discourage this patient from making any so-called affectionate advances toward the female technologist.

If an intoxicated male patient is radiographed by a male technologist he may tend to be abusive, using foul language and being generally uncooperative. If a female technologist is brought into the room these patients tend to refrain from such actions out of respect for the female sex. This is by no means standard behavior, but there is a tendency in this regard. You will need to adjust to the situation as you encounter this particular type of patient, but the presence of individuals of both sexes usually has a controlling effect. The most important factor is to handle yourself in a professional manner and be serious about your work.

Then comes good jolly grandpa, highly inebriated and feeling frisky as a young colt. These young female students look pretty good to him and hands will wander. Even when in this state, maintain respect for your elders. Tell them that their behavior can only get you in trouble with your superiors and ask if they would want that to happen? If they persist in being unmanageable, call in someone to help you, preferably your instructor or someone who could perhaps teach you how best to deal with the situation.

The male students, on the other hand, may encounter some intoxicated females and these can get quite out of hand. They can be either hard to get along with, silent and moody, or careless and romantic. With any or all types you must be very careful in your professional conduct. If you get strict with them they can cook up any number of stories to get you into trouble. You must, at all times, be serious and strictly professional while working with intoxicated females. Be especially careful that you do not accidently expose them or touch them in any private area. Should the female patients make any advances toward you, ignore them and keep out of their reach. Other intoxicated female patients may be very suspicious of the male technologist. They may refuse to undress for an examination or may insist on being covered with any number of sheets, etc., beyond normal reason. In this case it is imperative that you are not alone in the room with the patient; always call in a female technologist, nurse or other female attendant. This will eliminate the possibility of any accusations being made against you.

Older female patients may get overly friendly but as long as it remains at this stage there is no harm done. Keep the conversation going and you will find that these women cooperate much better. You may find yourself being told all about their problems. If such is the case, everything they reveal to you is confidential, unless it would be of diagnostic value to the physician.

WEEPING. A weeping patient—male or female—is a problem that comes about once in awhile. To endeavor to stop the weeping would be a problem and you may just make the situation worse.

If you are doing radiography on this type of patient your best approach to the situation is to let them weep until they feel its time to stop. Go ahead with your work; get their cooperation as best you can. If they start talking to you about their problems, listen to them; if possible, lead the conversation to something more pleasant. Try to cheer them up if you can, but do not overdo it. If you overdo your cheerup campaign, you may just revert them back to their tears.

DRUG ADDICTS. The drug addict may also be an occasional problem to you. If he is in a withdrawal stage or needs another "fix" he will be shaky, demanding, unreasonable, and could easily become violent. Do not try to handle the problem by yourself; get help, preferably a doctor. The addict is unpredictable and you are not qualified to handle him.

INDECENT EXPOSURE. A problem of great importance in unstable personalities such as alcoholics, drug addicts, or mental conditions is that of indecent exposure either accidental or deliberate on the part of the patient. You must always be extra careful with patients of the opposite sex. During radiographic examinations take care to cover the patients sufficiently and be certain they remain so. Intoxicated patients may expose themselves due to accidental carelessness or may do it deliberately. If this should happen, maintain your composure and cover the patient. If the exposure should be accidental, the patient may accuse you of doing it. Patients under the influence of alcohol or drugs may imagine all sorts of things. If they should lodge a complaint, this must be considered by your supervisors. This complaint will not necessarily be believed unless it happens more than once, and depending upon the particular patient. Regardless of the validity of the complaint, no technologist can afford having this type of complaint made against him. Therefore, again this advice, cover your patients well, even overdo it for the sake of the patient and for your own reputation.

Should patients deliberately expose themselves, often late in the day when a minimal staff is on duty, calmly cover them. Tell them in a serious manner to remain covered. Often a male patient may experience an erection while being radiographed by a female technologist. In such a situation, excuse yourself from the room and call in a male assistant. You will notice that the situation will have been quickly resolved.

Male technologists will sometimes be confronted by female patients who will try exposure or other methods to get them upset or aroused. They may try to expose their breasts or other parts of the female anatomy. If this female patient should invent a story or accuse you of anything, you will find yourself on the short end of the case. If it appears that you are going to encounter problems, call in a female technologist to assist you.

Society is composed of a wide variety of emotionally disturbed individuals. Sex is one of these weaknesses, so be aware of it; be prepared to handle the problem as it comes to you. At no time reveal to the patient that the situation upsets you. Maintain your composure and professional attitude, do not allow yourself to fall into any immoral thoughts or desires. Remember that these patients are ill and need help. Try to help them back to a normal level of human behavior; do not weaken and fall into their category.

CHAPTER XII

PROFESSIONAL HANDLING OF PATIENTS AND CONDUCT UNDER CERTAIN CONDITIONS

W E are now going to dwell on the patient as we encounter him in different moods and types of behavior.

A technologist may be an absolute genius technically, but he may also be an absolute failure in the art of human relations. When we deal with people who are ill, we must not think of them just as "someone to be radiographed." They are people— just as we—as good or better than we are, and subject to all the human feelings and emotions. During illness these feelings and emotions are magnified and intensified. We, as professional medical people, must be able to act as a stabilizing factor and guide these people to a more stable outlook. We will handle many patients in any one day and each of these will pose his own particular problem. In the first few words that we exchange with patients we will have to determine how to handle them, and all of them will be different. We will have to know how to converse and conduct ourselves in the presence of patients.

During the author's years of teaching he has seen some excellent technologists and many whose capabilities were questionable. After studying many of the questionable ones, he is led to believe that few of them were poor technically, but that they were poor in public relations. Patients are sometimes worried, tense, irritable, and simply "difficult to get along with." As professional people, we must be of a special breed—understanding and kind.

In our present day the cost of medicine and medical care is markedly increasing. Financial worries are great, for the patient may not have sufficient or any medical insurance. The days of Florence Nightingale are in the past. Very little of hospital work is voluntary but is paid for by the patient, or taxes. One thing we must always retain from the days of Florence Nightingale is our devotion to duty.

In the following pages let us discuss briefly some of the major technologist-patient relationship problems you will encounter. There are innumerable circumstances and situations and we could not begin to talk about all of them. It is hoped that these examples will give you a guide and motivate you to try to solve these problems by yourselves or with your instructors.

Conversation

First of all, let us discuss conversation. This is our means of communication with the patient and is of utmost importance. The tone of our voices relates our mood and how we feel. The tone of one's voice can say many things: "Why must I do this case?" "I'm not interested." "I'm late for coffee, already." "Gee, it's quitting time, and you had to come along!" On the other hand, it could say: "I'm glad to do your radiogram." "I'm sorry you're ill." "Get well soon!" We must have complete control over our voices, no matter how we feel or how trying the situation. Cultivate a voice that is always well modulated, sincere, interested, and kind.

Information you may unknowingly divulge is another problem. Patients are often clever in obtaining information from you by leading you on and asking simple questions. They may ask about their examination and what it usually reveals according to the symptoms that they have. Suppose you go ahead and tell them? The patients may arrive at many assumptions and become extremely upset about "the disease that they think they have." With many patients it is a good idea that they understand the examination, but you are not qualified, nor do you know enough of their past or present state of health, to tell them anything. Do not just avoid their questions; explain to them that their personal physician is the individual to tell them all about what they do or don't have. By pretending to be a highly intelligent, informative hero and telling them a lot that may not pertain to their particular case, you can cause them a great deal of unnecessary worry because of the conclusions they may draw.

In our work we meet many personality types; they are interesting as well as puzzling in the situations they create.

THE OVER-TALKATIVE PATIENT. Of these, we will meet many;

they will carry on a conversation as constant and rapid as automatic gunfire. In such a situation, never show irritation or impatience. You may inwardly wish these people would stop talking, but, remember, they are behaving this way for a reason. These people are usually nervous, high-strung individuals. Their constant chatter is a form of release for this nervous tension. They could be ill at ease and hoping to gain your friendship by talking. You must remember that perhaps the situation they are in is new and frightening to them. The sight of so many professional people, all dressed in white, may appear quite menacing and they fear what they do not know. Perhaps this is just their nature and they must talk a lot. On the other hand, they may have an ulterior motive. They may want to confuse or impress you so much that you will reveal the results of the examination. Perhaps they want you, as a friend, to give them a cut-rate on the charges for the examinations. No matter what their reasons are, we must tolerate them and handle the situation as best we can.

The question is, just what do we do or say in such a situation? Ignoring them will accomplish nothing except hard feelings and a poor reputation for the department. Common reasoning forbids our telling them to not question us—although we might feel like it. The old saying is, "if you can't beat them, join them." If these patients want to talk their jaws off, let them; answer them as the conversation demands. Remember one factor, however, do not make a social afternoon out of it, you have many other patients to attend. Do not allow yourself to be distracted so that the quality of your work will be affected. By treating the patients with respect, you make them feel that they are not just "cases" or a "number" to you. They are human beings that need your help and need to feel that you are pleased to help them. Such a feeling makes them feel more secure in this strange, forboding place called a hospital. Psychologically, you have aided them immensely by being a pleasant individual they could talk to. Indirectly, you have aided in a great part of their recovery by giving them security. I will remind you again, however, to be careful what you talk about; do not inadvertently reveal pertinent medical information that is not yours to reveal.

We now come to another type of patient who may or may

not be overly-talkative, but who does have a hundred and one questions and expects you to answer them all! These questioning patients present a real problem. Their questions, as a rule, will deal directly with their ailments, the examinations, what they usually reveal and the results of their own radiograms. Many times the patients are adolescents, where curiosity is only natural. The questioning may concern other patients, other examinations you do, and numerous "curiosity questions." Again, this type of patient needs to be handled skillfully as problems could easily be created.

If the questions concern the equipment, you can probably answer them as far as your knowledge permits. A very common question is: "how much radiation am I getting; how dangerous is it?" Your only answer can be that the amount of radiation being received is negligible, as modern machines and methods have reduced it considerably in the past decade. You may say that the danger is nil because the type of x-ray beam used with modern equipment (high kilovolts peak and increased aluminum filters) is less harmful than it used to be. If the patients are those who have been reading all of the radiation scare articles and appear to have some knowledge of radiation, send them to their physician or the radiologist for more detailed explanation. Assure them that if their physicians had felt there was danger, they would not have requested the examination.

If the questions pertain to the cost of the examinations, refer them to the business office when their examinations are finished; explain that you do not take care of the billing.

There are many questions for which you will not know the answers. Do not be afraid to say so, then refer them to someone who does. Do not try to be a hero and give them answers that are not completely true just to save face! If questioning is such that it becomes unbearable or their questions are beyond the realms of ethics, you have every right to tell them, in a proper manner, that you are not allowed to discuss such matters. Explain that there are certain hospital rules and rules of ethics you must adhere to. Remember to treat all patients with respect, answer all questions courteously. Do not at any time show impatience or annoyance; try to answer what you can within the rules of ethics.

Frightened

Another type of patient we must deal with will be the frightened patients. These patients will fall into two categories: the frightened adult and the frightened child. The adults may not show their fears outwardly but will harbor them within themselves. They fear the examinations, they fear what the examinations may reveal. These patients should be reassured and calmed down by the tactful technologist. One of our greatest present-day medical fears is the fear of having cancer, and rightly so. If the patients fear the examinations, explain to them that these are frequently used; tell them the approximate number of films you will be exposing and what they must do to help you. Try to keep a cheerful atmosphere in the room and try in a subtle way to engage the patients in some common topic of conversation. Any subject will do along the line of sports, current events or local events. If they take part in the conversation, it may ease their tension somewhat and reduce their fears. If you recall, the overly-talkative patients used this outlet for relieving tension; the same method can be used for frightened patients. Often they may end up telling you what their fears are and you will be better equipped to handle the situation. You must be careful what you are reassuring the patients about, do not be so naive as to reassure them that they don't have cancer, for you do not know this. In the event that cancer was later confirmed you would have toppled all their faith in any member of the medical profession. Reassure them that the examinations are safe and that the doctors will inform them of the results as soon as they are available.

Worried

The worried patients are of a similar category but instead of being tense and jumpy, they will be quiet and thoughtful. Try to draw them out in the same manner as the frightened patients but be aware of one factor. If the patients do not respond after you have made your move, do not persist. Many times the worried patients will cheer up somewhat and you will have accomplished something important in the patient's program of treatment. As with all types of patients, keep the atmosphere in the department cheerful. You cannot expect any patient to be reasonably cheerful if all the technologists are moody.

We should not lead you to assume the idea that your patients should be gay and witty as if they were at a party. The idea is to try to have them reasonably relaxed and confident of your work. It is easy to see you will not be successful with every patient, that is too much to expect. However, if you can cheer up someone each day it will make you a better person.

Extrovert—Introvert

Now we come to two types of patients who are emotionally disturbed to some degree. These people are known as "extroverts" and "introverts" in psychiatric terminology. In this day of tension and fast living there are more and more emotionally disturbed people. We must know how to work with them effectively. It is not our duty to counsel them or cure them; we could not, even if we tried. The following paragraphs are not meant for technologists in psychiatric hospitals, as that is a specialized field in itself. We shall try to deal with patients we encounter in society that come to active treatment hospitals. Some of these may not be diagnosed, as yet, but the actions will be there.

An extrovert is one whose primary interest is in the outer or objective world, his chief concern being with social and practical affairs. Occupied with worldly activities, he shuns self-analysis or criticism. This type of patient will try to impress you with his self-importance and high ideals. He may criticize his doctor and state, "there is nothing wrong with me." You must be respectful and not contradict anything this type of patient says. Let his doctor resolve any such problem. Do the radiographs, explain that you are doing them at the request of his physician. The sooner you can get your work done and get this type of patient back to his room, the better off you are. Remember to humor these patients and obtain their cooperation. Limit your conversation, if such is the case, to requests of them in positioning and turning.

The introvert, on the other hand, is deeply concerned with the subjective world of the imagination and spirit for which reason he is a subject of self-analysis and criticism. His center of interest lies in his own mental life and not in his environment or other persons. The introvert is withdrawn, thoughtful and deliberate in making all decisions. He does not like exuberant amusements, stories of daring adventure or activities which call for feats of skill. You do not greet this individual with gaiety or laughter. Proceed with your work in a quiet, professional manner. If this patient wants to carry on a conversation, oblige him. Never criticize or oppose this patient either; try to win the patient's confidence.

There are many types of mental conditions but unless we work in a psychiatric hospital we will not encounter them. Perhaps you have been helped to realize that you will meet patients of many types, in many moods. You will need to treat each as an individual according to his own needs.

CHAPTER XIII

SPECIAL CONSIDERATION FOR PATIENTS UNDERGOING ISOTOPIC EXAMINATION

MANY departments of radiology now have a specialized department for isotopic procedures, and students will be expected to spend a portion of their training period in this work. In other centers, the isotope department is a separate entity in itself and training is carried on as a postgraduate program. In either case, the following suggestions may be applicable as you encounter your individual patients.

Isotopic procedures require that radioactive materials of different strengths and natures be injected into or taken orally by the patient. This procedure in itself involves a certain element of risk and creates a certain amount of apprehension on the part of the patient. The technologist must prepare the patient psychologically so that these fears do not reach unwarranted proportions. It is not necessary to go into all of the technical or atomic details of the procedure as to exactly what is happening within the patient's body. However, it is important, depending upon the patient's ability to comprehend, to inform the patient that you are attempting to determine the function of a certain organ or section of the body. It is essential that you explain simply some of the equipment and the resulting sounds that they will hear as they are being scanned for the extent of radioactivity. A layman's explanation of the equipment should reassure the patient that he is not being exposed to some experimental rather than a known and proven procedure. Isotopes are still a relatively new field and little known to the general public, so some doubt and apprehension can be expected.

Some isotopic examinations take a relatively long time and the patient must be positioned and remain fixed for the duration of the examination. Depending upon the age, anatomical area in question, etc., the patient should be either seated or reclining in the most comfortable position. The patient should be kept warm (covered), and if in a reclining position the lights should be dimmed to prevent a glare into the patient's eyes. The atmosphere of the room should be warm, cheerful and comfortable. Since the patient will spend long periods of time in a fixed position the time will tend to pass very slowly and become tiresome. Soft, tape-recorded music has been found to be comforting and serves to pass the time more quickly and pleasantly.

Your conduct and general attitude are especially important in handling these patients. You will need to reassure them by checking frequently on their comfort during the procedure or answer any questions that they may have. Do not tend to become indifferent and try to "sit out" the duration of the examination as long as the patient expresses no verbal complaint. There should be no interruptions from phone calls, as your entire time should be occupied in checking of the patient and the equipment. Telephone calls would be startling and distracting as would other personnel entering or leaving the isotope room. At no time should the isotope patient be left alone in the room while the examination is in progress. We are dealing with a radioactive material that is being counted and if the procedure is left unsupervised the patient will tend to doubt the accuracy of the results. We are dealing with a radioactive material, little known and understood but greatly feared by the general public. If we are to build up the patient's confidence in the value of the procedure and our capabilities in doing it, then we must devote our full attention to it.

Noise and conversations adjacent to the isotope room should be kept to a minimum. The patient lying quietly during the procedure will naturally become quite sensitive to the sounds around him. Loud laughter or talk will be annoying; conversations irrelevant to the patient may be misunderstood and applied to themselves. Discussions of the results of other similar examinations, and the indications of these results can be confusing and frightening when heard in fragments through a wall or partially opened door.

Because of the fact that isotopic procedures are relatively new, it is imperative that the personnel handle themselves confidently. Nothing can be more frightening to an already worried patient than to have two or more confused technologists trying to calculate or determine the next setting on the machine, especially if there happens to be a difference of opinion. The patient expects to be cared for by confident, competent individuals who can evaluate every problem rapidly and handle the situation in a professional manner.

CHAPTER XIV

SPECIAL CONSIDERATION FOR PATIENTS UNDERGOING RADIOTHERAPY

IN the care of patients undergoing radiotherapy the student radiologic technologist will be required to fulfill possibly one of the most demanding roles with regard to attitude, conduct, and self-control. The role that the technologist plays in creating an encouraging and comforting atmosphere is vital to the progress of the patient on the road to recovery.

Radiotherapy patients may have some form of malignant tumor or lesion in or on their bodies. By use of radiation energy, the radiotherapist is hopeful of arresting or destroying these undesirable cells.

You will encounter many patients, and their attitudes and general outlook on life will vary from one individual to another. As a general rule, these patients are worried; worried about the effect of this radiation energy on their body, worried about its effectiveness in destroying the malignancy and what their prospect for the future will be. Many of these patients will have a depressed, rather deflated outlook and their desire to overcome their problem will depend a great deal on the attitudes and outlook of the therapists who will carry out the treatments. A very great factor instrumental in the recovery of any patient is the "will to live." This "will" can be kindled and encouraged by a sincere and interested therapist.

The department will be equipped with numerous therapeutic machines varying from the small superficial unit to the "one million volt plus" therapeutic machines. It is essential that the therapist handle this equipment confidently to instill confidence into the patient.

Often the attitudes of the therapists or students who have worked with this type of patient for some time may gradually become one of indifference. This is a form of defense mechanism against personal involvement. This feeling will be conveyed to the patient who will sense a particular type of hopelessness. You must develop and maintain a flexible attitude to fit the psychological needs of each individual patient.

Your initial encounter with the patient will be in greeting him when he arrives in the department. Your greeting must be sincere, cheerful and interested. The patient may be very sensitive to the reactions of other people and will be looking to you for some sign of encouragement. An over zealous, exuberant greeting can serve no useful purpose and will easily be detected as a false front. The demands on personal self-control in conduct and attitude in the radiotherapy department are very great. For this reason many schools will not assign students to this particular department until the very latter part of their training program.

If the patient has come to your department for the first time, he should be instructed briefly in the procedure that is to follow, the equipment and what he will be expected to do to help in this treatment. If you can occupy the patient's mind and keep it off himself, it will make the procedure much easier and time will pass more quickly. Do not simply lead the patient into the therapy room and proceed with the treatment without proper psychological preparation.

When the radiologist or radiotherapist enters the room, introduce him, simply as a means to establish communication. Relate points relative to the treatment for confirmation by the radiologist, or answer any pertinent questions the patient may have. Have the radiologist answer questions beyond your capabilities.

One of the most common questions in social conversation is "How are you?" or "how do you feel?" This is about the most certain way known to start anyone off on a running commentary about their ills. With some patients it will serve as a practical and leading question; with others it will serve to focus their attention on themselves and arouse their self pity. Your most practical approach to conversation may be on topics of current interest, people, places or things. If the patient is in a conversational mood and offers cheerful topics of conversation, pursue them intelligently. If the patient offers the comment that he feels better, tell him that this is very encouraging and not unusual. If the patient should venture the comment that he feels worse or that he feels badly, accept the comment quietly and try to encourage the patient as much as possible. The results of radiotherapy sometimes are not evident for several treatments or may produce side effects which this patient may be experiencing. If the patient simply accepts the treatments as inevitable and shows no emotion whatsoever, try to draw this individual out in conversation and reactivate his interest in life.

One of your objectives in this department, as in any other, is to show individual interest in each of your patients. They are separate entities and have individual needs. Even though this patient may be your fifteenth or twentieth for the day, you must approach each patient with the attitude that he or she is your only and most important one, not simply a name or case number in a log book.

Though your patients in therapy have their particular ailment and treatment in common, their personalities and attitudes will vary with each individual and their particular approach to their own problems. You must be flexible enough to vary your approach to each patient according to his apparent needs. This is most difficult, even for the seasoned technologist. You must be encouraging to all to engage in the uphill climb toward recovery and an extension on the precious gift of life. There will be times that you may feel the therapy is a mere formality but you must never convey this attitude, for you could very well be mistaken.

Although their particular case seemed medically hopeless, some patients have made a next to miraculous recovery because of a positive attitude and intense faith. Each patient must be treated with the attitude that recovery is expected and this must be sincere. People facing death become very perceptive and should not be treated in a patronizing manner. Your approach, your attitude must be genuine, and you, yourself, must believe in what you are doing. On the other hand, build no false hopes in anyone with remarks that are not factual.

Another important factor in the treatment of the therapy patient is in your approach and attitudes towards the members of his family or friends. You must win the confidence of the family and encourage them in the validity of the treatment, since it is recommended by the physician and the radiotherapist. Frequently patients suspect that the truth is being kept from them but has been revealed to their family and will quiz them accordingly. It is important that the family also give the patient encouragement and support.

Inevitably you will be faced with the treatment of patients whose prognosis is terminal. You must be concerned with their variations in strength and associated pain from day to day. The only encouragement that you can give here is in the degree that treatment may alleviate pain. Although you cannot be your cheerful, smiling self in your own heart, you do owe the patient reassurance, interest and a genuine desire to help. Should this individual have a naturally cheerful outlook on life in spite of its problems, let this be your guide to maintain that same attitude. If the attitude is indifferent or depressed, try to make him as comfortable as possible and offer any honest encouragement that you can.

The psychological approach of the technologist to the patient undergoing radiotherapy would fill a volume, inasmuch as each patient has individual problems and needs. In our capacity as technologists we can only employ some basic principles and common sense, for we are not psychologists. The general atmosphere of the department should be quiet, pleasant and comfortable. Our attitude and conduct should be one of confidence and assurance; we must believe in what we are doing, its purpose and chances of success.

Many times you will see some of your patients slowly deteriorate before your eyes and expire because of the disease; you cannot help but feel some personal sense of loss. You will also be encouraged at the sight of patients who recover and return to live useful productive lives. The fact that we do have many successful courses of treatment is encouraging and a sign of progress. As time goes by and the science of medicine progresses, the ratio of success shall exceed that of failure in radiotherapy.

The factors mentioned here are very basic and designed to motivate your thinking before you, yourself, encounter therapy patients. It is recommended that each student first approach the chief technologist of this department and acquaint himself with his psychology in the treatment of these patients. You must be able to determine the needs of therapy patients and implement them much more readily than for your other patients. The psychological atmosphere of the department and attitude of the patient are an essential part of the treatment.

CHAPTER XV

PORTABLE RADIOGRAPHY

PORTABLE x-ray unit radiography is, as a rule, more difficult than radiography with conventional equipment. We must be aware of the need for an entirely different psychological approach to the patient. Patients for portable radiography are often critically ill or cannot otherwise be physically moved as it would cause further injury. Portable units are taken to the patient's room. The radiography is done while the patient is in his bed, and care must be exercised to move the patient no more than absolutely essential. These patients may be under sedation or semiconscious and if they see the portable radiographic machine coming at them, with little or no explanation, they feel as if it is the end of the line. Remember, therefore, to introduce yourself to the patients and explain the purpose of the portable examination, that it will eliminate the possibility of further injury if the patients were to be transported to the radiology department.

On occasion, patients have become very upset when a student did not explain the portable examination. The patient feared he was dying and about to enter the "pearly gates." It takes a great deal of explaining and convincing talk to calm these patients down. This can and should be averted. The comfort of our patients, mental as well as physical, is our prime concern. We should never cause them any extra distress. The patients should be made to understand that portable radiography is a modern facility, for the benefit of the patients who require its convenience and comfort.

Accuracy of Work

Portable radiography is more difficult than working with conventional equipment because the equipment is smaller; there is a line voltage drop and other technical problems. Your accuracy in judging techniques under these adverse conditions must be better to compensate for the fluctuating factors with portable equipment. One of the major problems that is found among staff and students in portable work is their technical judgment.

Unfortunately, much of the portable radiography done has to be repeated because of poor judgment in determining technical variations. We must be very careful in handling the patient and judging of techniques, for a repeat examination may be impossible due to the patient's serious condition.

Aid from Floor Personnel

If you come upon a case of which you are in doubt, call someone to help you; consider the comfort of your patient first. In doing portable radiographic work always make certain that you have sufficient, qualified help for putting the cassette under the patient, moving the equipment, positioning and holding the patient. This help should be from the nursing staff, who is familiar with the patient and his injuries or ailments. This will lessen the possibility of further injury to the patient.

An important factor to remember, when employing nursing staff members to help you with a patient, is to provide them with the proper protective materials for their hands and bodies; e.g., lead-insulated gloves and aprons to protect them from any scatter radiation from the patient. Since nursing personnel may not be familiar with the exact positioning required of the patient, instruct them first so that they may be more helpful.

Extremely Ill Patients

Portable radiography on an extremely ill patient should be done with speed, without sacrificing the technique or the comfort of the patient. To eliminate apprehension on the part of the patient you should explain simply what you are doing and why. Have a sufficient amount of help present to do the work as quickly as possible with the least amount of discomfort to the patient. The sooner that the radiogram is available for the radiologist to evaluate, the sooner the patient's physician is contacted, the sooner the treatments may be determined and put into effect to alleviate the discomforts of the patient.

Critically Ill Patients

A patient who has extensive bone injury should be moved as little as possible to prevent further injury. Be certain you have sufficient help available. Do your work quickly and accurately. Every time you have a repeat examination to do, you are adding to the inconvenience of the patient, adding pain to injury, exposing the patient to more radiation and delaying the diagnosis. If you do your work rapidly and with assurance, the patient will cooperate much better. However, if you maneuver idly, hesitate, and change your mind, you will only annoy and inconvenience the patient. Therefore, competent portable radiographic work can only be done by a technologist who is quick, accurate, and one who has the interest of the patient at heart.

Portable Radiography on Cadavers

In the process of doing autopsies in the morgue, the pathologist may require some portable radiographic work done for the purpose of localizing foreign objects or determining the type and/or extent of injuries. Although in some larger centers the morgue may have its own radiographic equipment, usually the portable equipment from the radiology department will be utilized. As a senior student, you may be confronted with the assignment of doing portable examinations on a cadaver. You will be expected to work as carefully and professionally as you would with a living patient. The technical changes are not that much different unless some of the organic tissue or organs have been removed.

Occasionally staff members or students will become excited or repulsed by the idea of radiographing a postmortem case. Others are drawn with curiosity by the gruesome circumstances surrounding the cause of death. As with any radiographic work, you are ethically bound not to make this work a topic of conversation, especially in public or within hearing of patients and visitors. If you do, you will be betraying a professional trust and could inadvertently be overheard by members of the family or friends. You must respect the rights of the dead as well as those of the living.

CHAPTER XVI

ETHICS AND CONDUCT IN PEDIATRIC RADIOGRAPHY

SOME of the most trying and difficult radiography you will be called upon to do is the radiography of children. Your patients will range anywhere from the tiny newborn to the uncooperative preschool child to wise but often frightened ten-year-olds and those who are older. Many of them will know better but will be uncooperative due to fear, and fear of the unknown. Often these fears have been instilled due to poor teaching on the part of the parents. Often, too, these children have been threatened with doctors and hospitals as a form of discipline or punishment. The reasons for fear are legion.

One of the most important factors you must understand about pediatric radiography is that it requires a great deal of psychology, as well as technical knowledge, in handling children during the procedures. A new student technologist may know the positions required for certain examinations but be completely unable to obtain a good radiograph. Before you try radiographing children it is advisable to observe the seniors and registered technologists doing examinations and ask questions about anything you do not understand.

Children up to one year are difficult to handle by virtue of their age. They will be frightened and will cry and kick to show it. These children will have to be held or restrained in position. The older children will have to be talked to and treated differently. First of all, try to get the child to communicate with you. Children seem to sense people who like them and will respond to them. On the other hand, they can also sense people who don't like them and can become quite upset. If possible, let the child pick "his friend" from the technologists present. The security and well being of the child are most important. It is quite interesting how well a child responds to a person who can temper authority with kindness.

In child radiography we use high speed screens, high milliamperage and kilovoltage equipment plus other devices which your instructors will demonstrate to you. One of our best trick methods is to attract the attention of children as they do in child photography. If their attention is engaged for a few seconds, so that they sit still for a precisely timed exposure, we can obtain a good radiograph. Children, by nature, are curious of all things and their eyes and ears catch everything. Therefore, their attention may be attracted by bright objects or toys waved suddenly in the air or by sounding a bell or horn. When their attention is attracted, make the exposure.

Many times you will be unable to attract the child's attention and the squirming and yelling will continue. The last resort is to hold the child in position, as still as possible. In doing this we must be extremely careful not to hurt the child in any way. Sometimes a child has been bruised by holding his arms or legs too tightly. If the child is struggling violently the limb could be severely injured. Many times a child being held had his head free and was injured by banging his head on the examination table. Therefore, it should be realized that many factors must be considered and many precautions taken. Your instructor will demonstrate methods in safely restraining a child.

The child one to two years of age is often known as the "tough rebel" in radiographic work. Here we have to contend with a relatively strong child physically, and one with no sense of reasoning. He can and will often fight you throughout the entire examination and have energy to spare when you are exhausted. Try to win his friendship if at all possible. If this method fails, he will need to be restrained. Try to do the examination as quickly as possible.

The two- to three-year-old child may be somewhat easier to handle, if mature for his age and depending upon the nature of his parental upbringing. Try to win his confidence and explain very simply that you are going to take some pictures of him. Show him the table where he will lie down and the button you will push, etc., to interest him in what is going on. Have a supply of balloons on hand and promise him one if he does what you ask. These children still have very little actual sense of reasoning so you may have to resort to physical restraints.

A point of very great importance must be discussed at this time. Always remember to have at least one or two assistants when radiographing a child. Too many people may frighten him but you should never attempt to do an examination by yourself on a small child. *Never leave a small child alone on a radiographic table even long enough to turn around.* He can roll over and off the table so quickly that it would be impossible to catch him. You could be charged with personal negligence and you would deserve it! *Always have someone actually holding on to the child.*

A child three to four years old is a little more socially inclined and able to understand more of what is going on. His cooperation can be elicited fairly easily if you approach him in the proper manner. Never deceive a child; rather try to get the child to trust you and like you. Explain simply what is going to be done so he will not be afraid of all the monstrous looking pieces of equipment. Again use the explanation that you are going to take a picture. Some children are just plain uncooperative. With them be stern but kind. In the event this doesn't work, restraint must be used.

The four-to five-year-old knows and understands a great deal, especially if he has been taught well at home. Explain simply and truthfully what you are going to do. The picture-taking game is still the easiest for children to comprehend. If the child has had poor home training or is nervous by nature and decides to throw a tantrum, then you must still be kind but firm. He may eye you as if you were public enemy number one, but a child responds to discipline properly given.

Children past the age of five years require the basic rules of good radiography. If the child is frightened, calm him before starting the examination. Children of this age have a sense of reason and can tell you what they fear. Explain things to them simply so they can understand what is going to happen. Have someone else or you, yourself, lie on the table demonstrating what he will have to do. Often their past experiences in a clinic or hospital may have been unpleasant and they fear the same will happen again. Often they are afraid that you are going to give them a "shot." You must understand these fears and always have patience with any child. Many thoughtless parents threaten their children that if they do not behave at home, they will take them to the doctor so he can stick them with a big needle. Parents who have trouble controlling their children threaten them with doctors, policemen, and so on. Some children are afraid to the point of hysterics because of things their parents have told them. At times, you will find that the parents may have less sense than the children.

Children from seven years of age and up are by nature a bundle of curiosity and full of questions. To establish a rapport with children of this age and relax them in preparation for doing radiographic examinations, engage them in conversation relative to their level of interest and activities. Ask them questions, not necessarily related to the examination or their ailment, but about school, the grade they are in, favorite sports, activities, etc. Usually youngsters will respond, relax and cooperate to the fullest extent. It is not unusual for them to express an intense interest in the equipment and the examination that they are having done. Relate to them according to their age and level of comprehension.

All children have a need to be recognized and understood as individuals. If they receive this treatment in your department they will return to the ward or home brimming with information and enthusiasm about their venture. The parents will, in turn, appreciate the consideration given their child and feel more secure in the work that was done for them.

Many children are just simply difficult to manage and cannot be reasoned with. In such a case you must be firm and take command of the situation. If they see you mean business, they usually will settle down. Never lose your temper no matter what situation arises. Perhaps you know he is really just a "spoiled brat" but under no circumstances do you ever strike or handle him in a rough manner. Children are one of God's most precious gifts to man; remember this always and you will know there must be a reasonable way to handle any and every situation. You will learn that radiographing children is an art and those who can do it are to be envied. They must be patient, quick to take advantage of an opportunity, have nerves of steel and have an honest love for children. It serves well to understand the mind of a child.

Parents

When children are in the hospital the parents will spend as much time as possible with them. Small children especially get very homesick and emotionally upset when separated from their parents. Out-patient pediatric patients will be accompanied by one or both parents, another relative or possibly even the sitter. In doing pediatric radiography you may find the parents are a greater problem than the children. There will be parents who yell at, threaten, or even spank the children if they do not cooperate. Often this only upsets a child more than ever. Then there are the parents who look upon you as the headman of a torture chamber and "how dare you touch my child?" More often, if the parent can come into the room while you do the examination, the child will feel more secure. The parent can usually be the one to hold the child in position. On the other hand, there are many children who cooperate much better when on their own and the parents remain out of the room. You will find that you must evaluate and judge the situation and decide on the plan to follow. Even so, you will probably be wrong on many occasions. A number of suggestions could be made pro and con on the idea of the parent being in the radiographic room. Here are a few situations that should be discussed with your instructors for their opinions, for they may not agree entirely with the following approach.

Experience has taught us that the parent should not remain in the room if the child is to have an examination entailing intravenous injection. No matter how well you handle the situation, the parent may become emotionally upset to see his or her child subjected to any pain, real or imagined. The child, sensing this, may become quite upset also. Another thing is that you do not need a sick parent on your hands, too. When the parent is waiting outside, be sure he is far enough away from the room so he does not hear the child cry. The crying will sound worse than it really is and the parent will imagine all sorts of terrible things that you have done or might be doing. If you can, send him to the coffee shop, reassuring him that his child will be well cared for.

If the child is in for a relatively simple examination, a sensible, calm parent will be a help. If the parent is high-strung and nervous or the pampering type, try politely to keep him or her out of the room. This type usually spells trouble.

Although it may sound cruel or unfair, for all practical purposes the parents should be out of sight and out of sound. Ask them to wait; approximate the time it will take and add a few minutes so they will not become apprehensive should it take longer than expected. Psychologically, it will be easier on the parents if you are finished earlier than they had anticipated. If you should be delayed, they may imagine something has happened to their child. If the parents should insist on being present in the radiographic room, do not argue. Always be courteous, pleasant and professional, never showing annoyance. Explain the procedure, what cooperation you will need of the child and how he is to be positioned. If the child must be bound to prevent movement of a certain joint, explain how it is to be done without discomfort to the child. You will find if the parents know what is to be done, often they will not insist on staying in the room. You may also explain that another reason the child is bound is to prevent repeated exposure to radiation of the child and the staff. Parents appreciate having the examination explained to them. With this knowledge they may be better able to explain to the child what is going to be done. If the parents cannot handle the child, then you may suggest that they leave the room. Some children behave much better for strangers. Never engage in a verbal disagreement with the parents, even if you know you are correct. He is their child and so theirs is the right to decide what is to be done.

Briefly these points have been presented, hoping to give you some ideas to work on. These are by no means "rules" to be followed. Child psychology is a field all of its own and we are only to learn a small part of it, mostly by experience. Your individual problems will need to be solved between you and your instructor, but it is hoped that you will use some of these suggestions as a guide.

As mentioned before, some technologists will be much more competent than others in the field of pediatric radiography. The requirements are knowledge of your work, speed, patience and a genuine love for all children. It is, in itself, quite a challenge and rewarding in its success.

CHAPTER XVII

KNOWLEDGE TO BE KEPT IN CONFIDENCE
REGARDING PATIENTS

IN the hospital the patient feels he is at quite a disadvantage. He must reveal many personal facts and it is a problem to him wondering if they will be kept inside the hospital and protected. This personal information will be given reluctantly unless the patient feels secure and confident in the personnel that care for him. It is our responsibility to keep all information about the patient strictly confidential. Patients will cooperate fully only if they trust us.

One of the first important factors we must not discuss, outside of reasons of study, will be the radiographic reports on the radiograms. Basically, the only people who should know the results are the radiologist, the patient's physician, and the patient, depending upon just how much the physician feels he should reveal. The technologists may read the reports in order to study the results and find how they may improve on their techniques in taking future similar radiographs.

Our first big test in keeping information confidential begins in our own homes. Our immediate families will undoubtedly ask us about the sick people, the different diseases and injuries we have encountered. You may think it is ridiculous that we do not even discuss our work with our own families. For practical purposes and to maintain the highest professional standards, this is the way it should be.

At no time should we ever tell anyone outside the hospital "anything" about our patients. Your parents may give you the first degree, but you should tell them that you feel your patients would not want to be discussed as a topic of conversation. They cannot judge your progress by how much you know about your patients. If your parents want to know the progress in your studies, have them talk with your chief technologist. He will be more than pleased to talk to your parents and tell them of your work.

It may appear harmless to tell your family that you radiographed a patient today that had an advanced cancerous lesion in the chest. You haven't mentioned the patient's name or age or revealed his identity in any way. Actually, indirectly, it is a gross violation of ethics and a breach of confidence regarding the patient's personal information. First of all, your parents and other relatives may think that all technologists, nurses, *et al.*, are free with any and all information about their patients. If at some time they are patients, themselves, they will trust no one and, consequently, will not cooperate. They will use your "fault" to judge everyone by. Suppose they tell everyone about it? Can you imagine the damage you have done to your profession?

Let us use another example. Suppose you tell your parents about an interesting case, no names or identity. A few days later your mother—like a lot of mothers—will tell her neighbors how well her son or daughter is doing. She will tell of what an interesting case you did the other day. At this point this seems harmless but, again, there exists a severe breach of ethics. These neighbors may become ill in the future. Do you suppose they will go to your hospital, so you can tell everyone you know what is wrong with them? Indirectly you are ruining the reputation of your profession, your department, and the institution.

Let us say that the institution is the only one in a small community. Your mother told a friend of hers that you told her the other day that you had radiographed a seventy-five-year-old lady. The radiologist diagnosed her's as a very rare disease. Your mother's friend may have a seventy-five-year-old lady friend that was in the hospital at the same time. Immediately she will put two and two together and may know of the patient's rare disease even before the patient. On the other hand, this may not be the same seventy-five-year-old lady. Now suppose your mother's friend goes running to her friend and asks her how she feels, inasmuch as she has such a rare disease? Can you see what a chain reaction you have started? How do you suppose the little old lady will feel? Does she have the disease, or doesn't she? Think of the worry *you* have caused!

Do you now realize just how important it is to keep everything about your work in the strictest confidence? Not even the ones nearest and dearest to you can be told. Just tell them you are doing well; your work is most interesting and you hope to find success in your profession. Explain to them why you cannot talk freely about your work.

Your high school or college friends may ask you about your work. Tell them all about the subjects and courses that might interest them. Never try to impress them by telling them of the real "gory" examinations you may have done. You can be certain they will repeat your story, magnifying and distorting it at each telling. If they are interested in the course, send them to your chief technologist or school director.

You and your colleagues may discuss patients for study purposes within the confines of the department or classroom only. Once you have properly completed an examination, your work is finished. The rest is up to the radiologist and the patient's physician. The identity of your patient should be forgotten once your work is finished. Many times students have been heard discussing their cases and patients during coffee breaks or lunch time. Coffee time is provided for your rest and relaxation; at lunch time you should relax and enjoy your food; discuss outside interests.

Different hospital personnel may confront you about a certain patient or case. As a student, you have no rights or learned ability to discuss a case on a professional basis. Send this individual to your superior and let him handle the situation. Never indulge in "loose talk" about your patients when in the hallways; you never know who will hear, and what a poor impression this makes. Your best bet is to keep your mouth closed and eyes open—watch and learn.

Social gatherings often lead to discussions in medicine, hospitals, and finally the patient and radiologic examinations. Attention will be focused on you. Are you going to play the big hero and start revealing information that should be kept confidential or are you going to be a humble devoted technologist and change the subject?

If you are old enough and at a party, a couple of cocktails may loosen your tongue. One must have a lot of self-control to keep amusing or interesting facts to himself. Such a person is deserving of admiration!

Your biggest quizmasters will be the patients themselves. They will ask you all about their radiograms and reports. Some will resort to all sorts of trickery to get information. Naturally they are concerned about the results of their examination and want to know them. At no time do you ever divulge the results of the patients' examinations to them. This is up to the physician or the radiologist only. Patients have been known to call up the department and say that they are "Doctor X" and ask to have a certain patient's report read to them. If you are in doubt about the voice, do not read the report without proper verification. Refer the call to the chief technologist and let him handle it. If you are alone, ask the person to leave his telephone number and you will call back as soon as you have found the filed report. Check the phone number against your telephone list and see whether they correspond.

Many types of approaches will be used by the patients. Nevertheless, the radiograms and reports are hospital property. Very often the patients ask to see their radiograms or even want to take them home with them. They feel that if they have paid for the examination they are entitled to the radiograms. You must obtain definite permission from either the patient's physician or the radiologist before you allow the patient to view his radiograms. Never be talked into doing something you know is ethically wrong just in order to be a "good guy."

Frequently the physician will not show radiograms to the patients for psychological reasons. To a nervous, worrying type of individual a small fracture will appear much more serious. He may worry about this injury long after it has healed. Most radiograms will not reveal anything so evident to the untrained eye and the patients may imagine they have seen all sorts of deformities or tumors. Imagination can play many tricks and cause the patient a great deal of unnecessary worry.

Personal Opinions

In your two-year training program in radiologic technology you may radiograph approximately three thousand patients. In this group of patients you will encounter numerous different personalities. Many of these people you will like instantly; others you will dislike. This is a problem you will need to learn to control. You must never draw immediate conclusions; they may affect the quality of your work.

Every intelligent individual will form opinions about people, but as professional individuals we should not discuss these opinions with anyone. We are trained to handle all types of patients. Do not lose your self-control and display anger or displeasure with any patient. You must be in control of your voice and facial expression. You must maintain a smooth, pleasant, stable approach to all patient situations. Although you may not be aware of it, the patient is keenly aware of your attitude. Remember that individuals who are ill are not on their best behavior. You are not in a position to judge or criticize the actions or motives of others.

Conduct of Patients

The conduct of patients, no matter how amusing or ridiculous it may be at times, should never be a topic for gossip or conversation. People coming into the hospital for treatment may not be responsible for their actions. They may be under the influence of sedation, alcohol, emotional distress or extreme pain. You, as a technologist, must adjust to all these situations and handle the patients to the best of your ability according to what the situation demands. A patient's actions may be discussed with the chief technologist, the radiologist or the attending physician. You may learn from their opinions; they, in turn, may benefit from your information in reaching a diagnosis.

Background of Patients

In our work we will learn the background of many of our patients. This history will include past medical, social, financial information. In past experiences you may have noticed that "money talks." Will you be a victim of this fallacy and cater to the more wealthy, socially prominent, than to the social welfare patient? It may be quite a temptation at times but actually you will not have gained a thing. They aren't going to make you rich or lead you into their own social circles. You must treat all your patients with equal respect, each according to his need. The fact that a person is rich or on welfare is confidential information, not yours to discuss or divulge.

History of the patient's past ailments is most important to help diagnose the present ailment, for those ailments may be contributory. Sometimes this past history may not be totally reputable; however, we should not set ourselves up as judges of anyone else's character. Suppose one of our patients had been treated for alcoholism some years ago; that does not make him an alcoholic today. People are known to reform, so any past history should not influence our thinking.

Suppose one of our patients has had prior treatment in a mental institution; this does not mean he is still emotionally unbalanced. Our job is to do good radiography, not try to determine a patient's character. On occasion there may be past information about the patient that could be of diagnostic value; report this to the radiologist and consider your duty done.

Wealthy or socially prominent people often have a tendency to be more demanding and request extra service; nevertheless, if your work is always of the highest caliber then continue as such. Do not be influenced by the "almighty dollar"; it is something we can't go to the grocery store without, but it isn't our only requirement in life.

Any and all personal information should be kept in the strictest confidence. None of this information should influence our attitude or treatment of the patients. It can be discussed with the chief technologist, the radiologist or the attending physician, only inasmuch as it may help interpret the radiograms or shed light on past physical and mental conditions which may be contributory.

CHAPTER XVIII

KNOWLEDGE TO BE KEPT IN CONFIDENCE REGARDING THE DEPARTMENT OF RADIOLOGY

PEOPLE have one common weakness and that is to talk about each other. It takes a great deal of self-discipline to refrain from it totally. As you work day after day with your colleagues you will find them to be of different personalities. No matter where you go or what you do, you will meet with similar problems and personality clashes. You must learn to cooperate with all of them and cope with all situations.

As we work with these people remember that there are many personal things you will know and must keep confidential. Most of the practical work you will do together. They are all in training as you are, trying as hard as you are to learn the most and do their best. Like yourself, everything they do is strictly confidential outside the department. Some of your classmates may not be doing as well as you are; therefore, you should not discuss their progress with anyone. Worry about yourself and your own progress. If others are doing better than you, do not get jealous or try to ruin their reputation by spreading gossip. This only identifies you as a trouble-maker and no one needs you.

People may question you concerning your classmates, their progress, their personalities, their work or other information. At no time should you submit such information to anyone; let them ask the individual in whom they are interested. When you are a radiologic technologist and have responsibilities to the staff you may need to make out efficiency reports. These reports should be unbiased, impersonal reports true to fact. Personality differences should not influence decisions or reports on other employees. This is not a duty of the students, so adhere to your own rules.

As you finish your probation and become a junior student you may look at the senior students with envy. Never let your envy cause you to gossip about or criticize them. If they were not capable students, they would never have reached this stage of training. Observe them, respect them, try to be as good as they are or even better, but do not criticize or talk about them.

Instructors are always good material for student gossip sessions and disregard of rules of ethics. Being an instructor for some years does not necessarily indicate that this is condoned. Instructors have more responsibilities than are apparent. They are the tools that will mold you into radiologic technologists and most of the time this is not an easy task. These people will use many tactics to present the various subjects to you. Much of the time students do not realize or understand the true feelings of the instructors and how hard they try to get you to learn your subjects well. There seems to be a traditional feeling among student technologists that if students do well, then they are good students; if they do poorly, then the instructors are the ones to blame. Spreading stories about how poor the instructors are or that you are not learning anything will not get you "off the hook" in respect to your grades and practical work. Never try to degrade your instructors. If you are having problems with your studies, do not blame the instructors; discuss your problems with them and arrive at a solution. Talking things over with your instructors will dissolve your problems, but breaking the code of ethics and talking about your instructors can only harm you!

If you should be questioned about your instructors, you should have praise for them. If you have doubts about the instructors, approach them or the chief technologist personally, not the other personnel. Everything about your instructors should be confidential. If they truly were not qualified, their superiors would know and realize it. Degrading your instructors also degrades you and your school.

In the eyes of students, the chief technologists are always "mean" characters. Actually they are the most sincere and devoted of all. They have a great responsibility to the department, the registered radiologic technologists and the student technologists. These individuals must be concerned with having a department that is efficient, producing quality work, serving the patients well and maintaining a professional atmosphere. Any complaints you may have should be aired directly with them, not the rest of the world.

The radiologist is the director of the whole department and has a tremendous responsibility to his profession, the hospital, and his staff. There are many things about the radiologist that you will not understand. Do not reveal and discuss these matters with everyone you talk with. Ask the chief technologist and he may be able to explain all you need to know. Criticizing the radiologist simply because you do not know anything does not make you any better or him any worse, but it could do a lot of harm generally.

The radiologist is a doctor of medicine, specializing in the field of radiology. He is wise in the ways of his profession and what is best for the department. Although the rules of his department may be binding upon you, obey them. As you become more learned and more experienced, you will understand and appreciate them better. The radiologist's personality may not appeal to you or you may feel he treats you with indifference. What did you expect? Until you prove yourself worthy professionally, you are still nobody. Your life in the hospital has to be molded into a certain pattern different from that of your home life. You will adjust and grow into a mature, intelligent adult to make you better equipped in your profession. The radiologist is aware of this and tries to guide the teaching program to your advantage. The private or social life of the radiologist is also none of your concern. His higher standard of living was accomplished through hard work and he deserves it.

One situation that should not be tolerated in the department of radiology or the training school is the tendency for students to form cliques. Invariably the situation will arise where these groups will tend to criticize each other, the school, and the department. Such behavior is not conducive to maintaining a professional atmosphere.

If any of you determine that you like the profession and wish to pursue it further but cannot get along with your superiors or that you do not like the institution, then apply for a transfer.

This is much more constructive than venting your feelings to everyone you meet and criticizing whomever or whatever you are not in agreement with. There is nothing more destructive to the spirit of a group than to have someone continually complaining or criticizing. The chances are very good that if you cannot adjust to the individuals in this department you will have the same problem wherever you may go. You should discuss your problem with a school official in whom you do have confidence and trust, and arrive at a satisfactory solution. Anyone who finds himself in a situation not to his satisfaction will invariably find it difficult to refrain from divulging information that should be kept confidential.

CHAPTER XIX

KNOWLEDGE TO BE KEPT IN CONFIDENCE REGARDING THE INSTITUTION

W E have already discussed the institution and how it functions. Let us now consider some information about the institution that is confidential and should not be divulged. Exceptions are holiday parties, fund-raising projects, graduating classes of students, or events of public interest.

When patients are admitted to the hospital they will be asked for pertinent information. Information includes occupation, employer, religion, financial status, type of insurance. This information is strictly confidential and the patient's signature must be obtained before it can be released. Any information released without the permission of the patient could be grounds for a lawsuit. Remember, never be responsible for any leakage of information.

Some patients may be admitted and found to have positive tests for venereal disease or some other less usual condition. This information should not be used as food for gossip. Loose talk around the hospital is the worst menace that faces most institutions. When you have several hundred employees in an institution you are bound to have a few with big eyes and ears and bigger mouths. This type of individual should be dismissed from employment immediately. Unfortunately, this may not be discovered soon enough and much damage could result. Each employee in the hospital, directly or indirectly, helps the patient to get well. In order to do this efficiently, each must devote all of his time to constructive means and not in gossip.

In some years of experience one comes across people who work at a hospital or clinic, earn their living there, but still go around criticizing the place to everybody and anybody who will listen. Just remember one important thing about such a situation, if you can't say anything complimentary about your place of employment, "quit!" Obviously, if you are unhappy, then your work cannot be of the highest caliber. Complaining can only hurt your reputation and that of the institution.

If you should quit your training or place of employment, do not do so with resentment. This is a democracy and you are leaving the place of your own free will. If you were discharged then it must have been your fault and accept it as a lesson in life. Accept it as a correction and try to learn from it.

Many times individuals may come to our institution and immediately start to talk about their last place of employment. Mostly these facts are unfavorable criticisms. If you can't say something favorable about a place, then do not say anything. By criticizing, you are showing your ignorance and lack of ethical training.

Criticisms are also conversation topics among employees themselves. If you are dissatisfied about something, go to the personnel director or your immediate supervisor and discuss it with him in a rational manner. Discuss matters and this knowledge will make you a better employee. If matters cannot be explained to your satisfaction, "quit!" Constant gossip and complaining can only disrupt the atmosphere and harmony of hospital work.

In our professional society of radiologic technologists we will associate with students and radiologic technologists from other institutions. We will attend educational programs, conventions, and social functions. Even though we know that we never discuss our work on the basis of mentioning patient names, we can discuss the different techniques to be used on different cases. We will see displays of extraordinary radiograms and learn a great deal from them. Another factor may creep in on our discussions, and that is criticism of different institutions. All too frequently technologists have been known to criticize their own institution or school and complain they are hindered in learning their professional work. Never criticize your institution of training, even if it is not the most modern and up-to-date; remember, you chose it. If you can't say anything good about it, then "quit"; it doesn't need you. Professional people are ethically sound, responsible people and you must be equal to them. Remember that your school is accredited so it must meet the requirements established by national educational standards. The schools are evaluated regularly by appointed inspectors and their reports submitted. Therefore, your criticisms are unsound and display only your ignorance and poor judgment.

You will encounter students at various conventions, state and local educational meetings, etc., discussing either their own or other training schools. This can easily create dissention among the schools and spread to the graduate staff, even though such discussions would appear like a healthy attitude to take. Certainly schools can learn from each other's programs, policies, etc., but there are better channels to follow than the student "gab sessions."

If another school appears to be inferior to yours, do not make this a topic of humor. If, on the other hand, your school or institution appears to be inferior, don't complain; do something constructive about it. Approach the director of the school or the chief technologist and offer the information that you have. Schools are evaluated at regular intervals by qualified educators and certain standards are set for schools to follow. Be certain that any information or criticisms you have are justified.

Another frequent topic of conversation and dissatisfaction is the stipend that students receive during their training period. This will vary from one institution to another and the amount is no indication of the qualifications of the school. If your intentions in entering training at a school are determined by the amount of stipend rather than the school's reputation, then your philosophy for entering radiologic technology is slightly distorted.

In summary, if you cannot support your school, the institution, your instructors, etc., then determine the cause of your doubts, discuss them with the proper, qualified officials and arrive at a conclusion. If you cannot solve the situation satisfactorily, then it is time for you to move out into more compatible surroundings.

CHAPTER XX

KNOWLEDGE TO BE KEPT IN CONFIDENCE
REGARDING ATTENDING PHYSICIANS

PHYSICIANS are highly learned professional men in their respective fields, but, being human, they are subject to all human errors and weaknesses. Some physicians are better than others; some are specialists in certain fields of medicine and better than their colleagues in the same field. However, we must remember that they are all qualified men or they would not be allowed to practice. By observing many doctors you may form personal opinions with regards to their apparent professional knowledge, personal attitudes, doctor-patient relationship, etc. However, at no time are we qualified to be able to rate one physician as "good" or another as "poor." Remember at all times that any physician in practice has been passed by the Board of Examiners of the American College of Physicians and Surgeons. They must certainly be qualified before being allowed to carry on a practice. Omit forming opinions of physicians, lest they begin to show outwardly while working with them. Do not become overly-friendly either, for you could make a nuisance of yourself. Some physicians may treat you like a buddy, but, remember your place and continue to treat them with respect. Any show of disrespect or displeasure while working with a physician will result in immediate dismissal from training. You should devote your time to help all physicians to the best of your ability.

In various types of emergencies and examinations, the doctor may express different attitudes towards his patients. At times he may display a sympathetic attitude or a strict attitude, perhaps fatherly, or varied attitudes as would seem to fit the occasion. His attitude may be a form of psychological therapy to win the confidence of his patient, or perhaps he is aware of the patient's emotional stability and has a purpose for his action. Regardless of what the attitude is, at no time should you question the doctor, his patient or their relationship. Many times it may appear that the doctor is being pushed around by an over-demanding patient or that he is overly-friendly with the patient. He understands the patient's needs and meets them with the best psychological approach.

At first contact with a patient, the doctor may question him with regards to past medical history, present illness and personal problems at home or at work. As radiologic technologists, we should never divulge any information given in our presence. If any of it will help us in our work, apply it as such; otherwise, "forget it" for it doesn't concern us. The doctor is relying upon our ability to keep professional confidences.

Results of examinations upon the patients are most confidential. Often you will assist the doctor or radiologist in examinations and they are the only persons with whom you may discuss the resultant radiograms for learning purposes. The patient relies upon you to protect information private unto himself and discuss it with no one outside of your line of work. If you find it difficult not to discuss and reveal information regarding patients to your friends or family, then quit your training! You are in the wrong profession. You may do someone irreparable harm with your big mouth!

As you work day by day with different doctors you will form opinions of them as people, as doctors, as learned professional men and women. You must learn to work harmoniously with them at all times in a professional atmosphere.

Doctors, as people, have personal habits, too. Faults such as cigar smoking in front of a sick patient or coming to see a radiogram with liquor breath should not influence us too much. This should not be food for gossip, either in the department, hospital, or outside. No one is perfect; neither are you. If at any time you think you are faultless in your work or conduct, then you are not human. If anyone should ask you for your personal opinion of a doctor, tell him that he is a capable man, he must be if he is in active practice.

Doctors are frequently active in civic and social affairs, and, as a rule, well-known. You will meet the doctors at sports events, social, or public functions. The question will arise of how to speak to them and what to talk about. First of all, you never discuss hospital work or their patients. For example, if you are at a football game, discuss football; form your conversation around the event you are attending. Show them the professional respect due them and refrain from medical subjects. If you should belong to the same club, treat them as fellow club-members, but, remember, do not carry this attitude over to your hospital relationship.

Many times the doctors hold important official positions in different organizations in society. The doctor will never take his outside activities to the hospital and neither should you. His outside life is his personal business and should not influence his work professionally.

As soon as you commence your training you will have friends and relatives ask you which doctors are the best and to whom should they go with their ailments. This could be a tough decision. You could use your personal opinion but this is not always advisable. Rather than naming only one physician, name several and let them make their own choice. If they ask for a specialist, name several, and mention that they are all considered "tops" in their respective fields. In this manner you will at no time be soliciting for any particular doctor, for it would not be ethical. Let people make up their own minds.

One should remember that everything the doctor does for the patient is confidential; all information is pertinent, be it actual information or personal opinion about the doctor, and must be treated as strictly confidential.

CHAPTER XXI

CONSIDERATION FOR RELATIVES OR FRIENDS OF THE PATIENT

DEPENDING upon the location of your department within the institution, you may encounter visitors who have become lost while seeking someone that is a patient in the hospital. The patient may not be in the radiology department; the visitors may not know which floor he is on or may have no idea where this particular floor is.

On an extremely busy day, the natural tendency would be to ignore or avoid queries from these individuals. However, these persons are very important to the patient and, therefore, important to the institution. Every student and every employee of the hospital has a certain responsibility in promoting the public relations of the institution. The general public is entitled to a certain amount of courtesy and respect and should be assisted in every way possible. To the patients, their relatives and friends, the hospital is often a depressing and gloomy place and possibly the source of unpleasant memories. Even though you may be very busy when someone asks a question, take some time out to help him or else direct the inquiring person to the source of the information needed. It is true that your first responsibility is to the patients and not to run an information center. However, the visitors will relate to the patient the treatment received at your hands. Should that patient need to have radiographic examinations done later, you may get the same cooperation you gave his family or friends. If you were courteous and helpful, the visitors will encourage the patient with reports on the department and the institution, and he will feel more confident about his care.

Relatives

This particular section relates to the relatives who usually accompany out-patients to the department. Although the patient is your major concern and you will be directing your efforts in his behalf, do not forget to recognize the needs of the family. Be pleasant and courteous. After all of the information has been obtained from the patient with the help of the family when necessary, you should then take time to direct the family to a comfortable waiting room. Inform them of the location of the restrooms, concession stands, lunch room, etc.

Inform the family of the expected length of time that the examination will take. Be certain to allow time for repeats, etc., should the need arise; this will alleviate anxiety on the part of the family should it take longer than expected. Even if you need to take extra time, you may be finished before the time you specified to them, which will be a psychological relief to those waiting.

Be particularly wary of any information you may inadvertently divulge to the family through answering seemingly harmless questions. Do not be taken in by a lot of questions, answering them and revealing information only the physician has a right to divulge. In the event that they press you for pertinent professional information, refer them directly to the physician or the radiologist.

The Very Anxious Relative

There are relatives that may come in who are extremely anxious to see the patient (e.g., parents coming in after an accident in which their child was involved). Relatives closely associated with the patient may display a great deal of anxiety concerning the condition of the patient and demand to see the patient immediately. Such a situation is very tricky and you will need to handle it quickly and tactfully. Since their presence in the room might interfere with emergency measures, quickly seat them in the waiting room and inform them that you will talk to the doctor and tell him that they are present. It is imperative that you notify the attending resident or physician that the parents or family are present. The physician will then determine whether the family may see the patient or what information he wishes to relate to them. In such a situation it is important that you, yourself, do not relate any information as it may not be accurate. Injuries are frequently deceiving to the person who is not capable of diagnosing their extent.

Even a few abrasions which have been bleeding may present

a picture more severe than what it actually is. On the other hand, injuries may be camouflaged by clotting, hair, etc., and be more severe than apparent. To the unskilled individual, the sight of the patient may be upsetting and very traumatic. Leave the duty of diagnosing and reporting to the family to the physician, who is qualified and responsible.

The family or friends of the patient are of major importance and should be treated accordingly. If you are their first contact, make the information they desire available to them through the proper channels. Show them the same consideration you would wish to have in a comparable situation. Depending on the circumstances surrounding the situation, the family may require supportive measures and you may be the only one free to give it to them. Be pleasant, courteous and helpful.

Law Officers Investigating

A high percentage of the radiographic work done in the department will be on accident victims. The personnel in the department will come in contact with law officers either accompanying or following up these accident cases, and it will be expected to cooperate with the police department as requested. The department must accord the law enforcement officers courtesy and respect and assist in directing them to obtain information from the patient, or the family if present. If the patient is conscious, coordinate, and awaiting his turn to be radiographed, allow the officers to get their work done first; if the patient is being radiographed, inform them immediately when the patient is free for questioning.

Law officers have a public duty and trust; you may be present when confidential information is related to them. It is your responsibility to keep this information in confidence unless it has some diagnostic value. If you are in possession of information that may be helpful to the law officer you should relate it to him, and he will confirm it with the patient or the family; in this you have fulfilled a civic duty. The officer will determine if it is of value in the performance of his duties.

In summary, afford the law enforcement officers your full cooperation. They are performing a duty which is to the advantage of all citizens and are worthy of our trust and confidence, courtesy and respect.

CHAPTER XXII

FRIENDS, RELATIVES, HOSPITAL PERSONNEL, PHYSICIANS AND/OR THEIR FAMILIES

W HEN it comes to doing radiography on a friend or relative, we find that we have a new set of problems and must follow a particular pattern in solving them.

Let us first discuss the relative, e.g., a cousin or an uncle. Doing radiography on a close relative poses many problems and one of them is modesty. A person unknown to you may feel more at ease. This patient displays varying degrees of modesty but this can be met by proper draping and covers. A relative knows you and you may have many of the same friends. The situation of having to undress and be covered only with gown and sheets while you proceed with the examination may be disturbing. In focusing for the examination, you will need to locate various prominences by feeling for them. In the future you will be in the home of your patient and vice versa, and your relative-patient may fear that you will make some comment about the examination. He may not realize the factors involved in professional ethics and that you are bound by them never to discuss your patients in public. Remember your professional conduct applies to each and every patient, no matter who he or she may be.

Another factor we have to consider is that a relative may feel you should not charge him for the examination, or, at least, give him a discount. Relatives may become insulted if they are charged the same as everyone else. The only thing you can do is explain that you have no control over the charges or billing. Ethically, you have no right to do free radiography for anyone unless specified by the radiologist or the hospital.

Another problem that occurs with some relatives is that they will form opinions of your capabilities, conduct, knowledge, etc., when the examination is performed. There is nothing worse than having some aunt or uncle go around and tell all about the errors you made in the examination. It may be just your luck that a very common error could occur in the examination because you were tense or tried extra hard to do well. And, of course, dear relatives will capitalize on your misfortune and exaggerate it just a little. They may want to know how well you are doing in your training. This information can come from your parents who will have received it from the training school and no one else.

A problem that may come up is that relatives will not want you to know the diagnosis. They have no control over this as you have access to the radiograms and/or reports. On the other hand, they may insist that you tell them the diagnosis; this is not up to you but to their personal physician. Simply explain that ethically you can tell no one about his diagnosis and that you are not trained to interpret the reports. This can only be done by the physician or the radiologist. Relatives may hold a grudge momentarily but if they are reasonable people they will respect you for keeping information confidential.

Radiographing a close friend poses much the same problems as that of a relative. This friend may be one from your school days who perhaps has not progressed as well as you thus far. Often your friends are your worst rivals and enemies if they can get something to hold over your head. They, too, may capitalize on your errors. Remember no examinations are done as personal favors, compliments of the house.

Now comes your part; never "show off" either for friends or relatives. Avoid doing radiography on them unless it is necessary. Do not try to prove your knowledge or capabilities by outward demonstration. If you are a capable, skilled student technologist it will show up in the quality of your radiograms. Your reward should be self-satisfaction and pride. If you are a good technologist it will show without your campaigning about it.

Radiographing members of your immediate family should be avoided entirely unless you are the only one available to do it. There will be an emotional factor involved which could be hazardous in the lines of good judgment. You could be upset because of outside factors associated with the reason for the radiography. Let some other technologist look after your immediate family.

Your presence may be more beneficial just to stand by and comfort or talk with them. There will no doubt be exceptions to the rule but in the interest of better judgment, let someone else do the examination.

Many times other hospital personnel will require radiographic examinations. Some of these will be on an out-patient basis, others as patients in the hospital. Whenever you do radiography on the hospital personnel, do it with the most professional attitude of which you are capable. Maintain this attitude throughout the entire examination. Never comment on their examinations to any other hospital personnel or anywhere else in the hospital or out, jokingly or otherwise. They are entitled to your professional confidence as well as anyone else. Also, they may insist on knowing the results, which you are obliged not to discuss. As always, revealing the results is up to the physician. Your professional conduct will be appreciated by the personnel if they know the results are kept in confidence and not broadcast over the entire hospital. It is a good practice never to be overly-friendly with other hospital personnel.

Occasionally we may be faced with the duty of radiographing colleagues from our own department. Under these circumstances the importance of minimizing the amount of radiation exposure should be emphasized. Secondly, your colleagues are to be treated with the same consideration and respect as every other patient; there should be no joking or "kidding around." Again, because of the fact that your colleagues are also very close friends, the examinations should be done by a technologist of the same sex. As to the results of the examination, diagnosis, etc., you are still bound by professional confidence. The diagnosis is not a subject for discussion or humor and is the private concern of the patient and his physician. As with all children and young people, special care must be taken in shielding them, especially the reproductive organs. In the case of student radiologic technologists, who receive a certain amount of radiation in the course of their daily work, exposure to unnecessary radiation must be avoided at all costs.

There will be times that the staff doctors or their families will require radiographic examinations. You may be called upon to do some of these examinations and, as always, your conduct should be exemplary. When you are doing an examination on a physician, he will expect your conduct to be above criticism. You must never, at any time, become familiar or casual with a physician. Treat him with respect as you do when he is on duty. Do the procedure quickly and accurately.

When working with members of the doctor's family, treat them with equal respect. They are familiar with professional ethics and conduct. Do not overdo it and try to impress anyone. You will be respected only if you behave in a friendly courteous, professional manner.

CHAPTER XXIII

PROFESSIONAL ADJUSTMENT

Cooperation with Others

IN the first few months of training, aside from the technical aspect, will come the problem of emotional adjustment. Within the small world of the hospital you will need to adjust to communicating with a large number of people. You will need to learn cooperation and professional conduct.

Your first and closest associates will be your classmates. Some of your questions may be: (a) Are they friendly and easy to get along with? (b) Can I work with them on duty? (c) Can they also become my social friends? Suppose we look at some of these problems and possible solutions.

Your work—training and studies—will be done as a class. You cannot isolate yourself and learn this work on your own. A student who can discuss, demonstrate, and debate in the proper manner (even though he may often be incorrect), is an individual who will learn and conquer. In any profession, in order to be successful, you must be able to listen, ask questions, express opinions, correct your errors, and apply yourself. It is not a recommended practice to form cliques within your group; you must work as an entire class. Cliques cause strife among classmates and are not conducive to good progress. Many times the better scholastic students may "stick together" and, likewise, the poorer ones. This is unwise and poor professional adjustment. It may show up in your practical work and be evident to the patient. Keep your relationship on an equal basis, help each other, discuss and solve the problems. Your progress should be unanimous as a class, take pride in it. Never allow personal jealousy or prejudice to interfere with your work. Do not envy the brighter student; study harder yourself and become an equal. This type of constructive competition will produce better end results. You are on your way to becoming an adult; act like one.

A large percentage of students of radiologic technology are recent high school graduates. In many ways they are immature and rightly so without professional training. Students will be of both sexes and here also is an adjustment to be made. There will undoubtedly be dating among students and this will lead to problems on duty. Students may start "going steady" and demonstrate their feelings while in the department. This type of situation cannot be tolerated as it is detrimental to the atmosphere of the department and will affect your work. You will have to work in teams with your fellow students in the darkroom, the different radiographic rooms and other rooms within the department. If your "steady" is your partner for the week, emotional matters could get out of hand and the results would be unfortunate. It wouldn't be the first or last time couples would be caught "necking" in the darkroom. The only alternative to such behavior is dismissal of both parties from training. It is a good policy to avoid personal relationships with departmental personnel, even with hospital personnel. Such relationships are not conducive to a professional atmosphere. Do not misunderstand: Dan Cupid is not opposed, but the concern here is with the patient, the department, the profession, and yourselves. Your reputation must be one of a level-headed mature individual, not a starry-eyed teenager. Your social life and your professional life should be two separate entities.

One of the big problems of the freshmen is the professional adjustment of controlling themselves in temper, conduct, and speech. In high school or college you may have been more carefree and outspoken. However, in an institution of professional people, you fall into a new adult category, a school of hard and fast rules. You are not allowed to display evidence of temper, no matter if you are correct and someone else is not. One has to be an even-tempered individual, able to accept both criticism and praise. You will not openly criticize your colleagues, particularly in front of a patient or doctor. Let the problems be handled by the registered radiologic technologists in charge of your particular room. Problems can be solved in a rational manner, at the proper time, in the proper setting.

Many times an individual is unconsciously a "loud" person.

He may be loud in his speech either near the patient or in the immediate vicinity of the patient. His general conduct may be loud or noisy. Around the department one must be a reasonably quiet, efficient worker; many patients cannot tolerate noise because of their illness. This trait can be overcome by self-discipline and concentration. Develop a professional attitude and learn to think and act in an orderly fashion. At the same time, you must maintain an atmosphere of quiet sympathetic understanding for the patient.

An individual who is overly quiet and reserved is also at somewhat of a disadvantage. This person displays little or no personality and may go about his work creating an atmosphere psychologically damaging to the patient. He may appear so moody or expressionless that it may appear to the patient that he—the patient—has no chance of survival. One must reach a happy medium of self-expression that has the most suitable effect on both patients and staff. Moody, quiet people are difficult to understand; loud people are hard to tolerate. The quiet ones may end up being ignored by the staff because of this trait. Any adjustment problems you may have should be discussed with your instructors. They will try to advise you to the best of their ability.

We could go on indefinitely on the subject of professional adjustment to medical work. The above brief explanations and examples will motivate your thinking and set you to analyzing yourself and evaluating just where you stand. A person of strong character and abilities has the foresight to criticize himself and see himself in the eyes of others. If you have problems, discuss them with your instructor, the chief technologist, or the radiologist. Together you can improve upon or eliminate undesirable traits. You must respect your colleagues and observe them. Always try to improve yourself, but not at the expense of others.

Invariably, freshmen students attach themselves to the senior students. The question now comes up, just what should be the professional relationship between the freshmen and senior students? Senior students are people hard at work perfecting themselves in radiographic work. They may appear to be ignoring you at times but they have already learned all the preliminary work and are busy polishing the edges and becoming more proficient.

Naturally, they leave all the teaching to the instructors but, since they must work with you, they will often explain certain procedures to you. Be in a position to accept the explanation, ask questions, and display a respectful attitude toward your older colleagues. Do not try to copy your seniors in a fashion that would be annoying; cultivate your own characteristics. In your association with the senior students try to remember that even though they are also students they are superior to you in experience and knowledge. There is nothing that irritates senior students more than a smart aleck freshman that tries to show up and degrade others. You can only harm yourself with this type of action.

Your immediate supervisors, the registered radiologic technologists, are probably your most difficult problem in professional adjustment. First of all, these people have a difficult job to do in supervising you. You, as students, come from all walks of life and possess a variety of personality traits. Some of these traits are unfavorable and must be changed if you wish to pursue a professional career. You should understand this and not obstruct or defy any disciplinary measures that the registered radiologic technologists must take. Do not harbor an attitude of dislike for them, because if you cannot respect authority you have chosen the wrong profession. Respect them, follow their orders and remember that they are bound to make technologists out of you; that is your purpose in being here. Do not let your personal dislike of any technologist become so strong that it will affect your work.

True to form, there are other students of an opposite nature. They will indulge in "apple polishing" or any other tactics at their command to further themselves, no matter who else they have to step on to do it. Any student of this type is a menace to the school, the patients, and the profession. This type of behavior lowers the standards of the school and its whole morale. Any registered technologist who accepts such an individual should also be dismissed from the department as he does not possess supervisory abilities or judgment. Professional adjustment to the instructors follows along a similar line as that of the registered radiologic technologists, plus extra added factors. The instructors are faced with an enormous task. They spend long and extra hours preparing lectures, classes, examinations and correcting papers. Instructors are cognizant of students who deliberately ask questions that are immaterial to the subject or the course. If the instructors were not qualified or capable, they would have been dismissed by their superiors. Perhaps you do not care for the material presented by the instructors but it is of value and necessary for you to learn. The instructors will usually try to answer any and all questions the students ask, because they feel this is a sign of student interest and they try to encourage this. Do not try to waylay or mislead your insructors, for any loss of material or time is your loss, not that of the instructor. The instructors have already learned all this material and you are fortunate to have them. Many of our present day radiologic technologists did not have any instructors and had to learn a great deal on their own, often from texts which were sketchy and incomplete. The instructors, it is reiterated, are here for your advantage and no one else's. Any display of deliberate disrespect toward the instructors should result in immediate dismissal from training.

The chief technologist has a certain amount of prestige in the radiology department. He (or she) has worked up to this position step by step and has proven capable of handling such a demanding job. The chief technologist expects to be treated with respect by the students and radiologic technology staff, and rightly so. Although policy may vary from one radiology department to another, you will find that you can not treat your chief technologist as you would a "pal." It would be necessary to discipline you when needed, and to praise you if praise is due. The department is only as good as the chief technologist who is running it. The chief technologist is directly responsible to the radiologist, who, in turn, expects the department to run in compliance with his request. The chief technologist enforces the rules and runs the department with an iron hand. If you have a goal to become a chief technologist, just remember that it takes a great deal of study, hard work, and determination.

The radiologists are specialists who have detailed knowledge of a section of medicine known as "radiology." The radiologists have technologists to help them in their work. They have chief technologists to supervise the departments and see that the quality of work is superior. All communications with the students will most likely be relayed through the chief technologists. The radiologists may conduct some classes but this varies from one department to another; they have instructors for the entirety of the student training. Your main contact with the radiologists will be when you assist in special examinations and fluoroscopic work. It is their desire that all students in their schools become top-rate technologists. They are to be treated with the respect due them as doctors and specialists. No undue familiarity with the radiologists will be tolerated at any time. Strictest professional ethics are to be maintained in the department at all times.

You will have many occasions to work with the personnel of other departments. Your association with them represents not only you but your department also. Surgery is one department in which you will do a lot of radiographic work. Be pleasant with the surgery staff, respect the doctors and follow the rules of technique required. Do your work to the best of your ability; speed and accuracy are essential. Maintain your friendliness on a professional basis. Remember, again, you are representing the radiology department and that is a great responsibility.

The medical laboratory department also has a large number of students. There will be interdepartmental friendships made and you must remember to maintain them on an adult and professional basis, while on duty in the hospital.

You must try to maintain a harmonious and cooperative relationship with all hospital personnel. Follow and respect the rules in the respective departments. Your ability to do this will determine the degree of your professional emotional adjustment. Do your work to the best of your ability. You will be put to the test many times, but at no time should you display temper, lest you only degrade yourself, your department and your profession. If at times the staff in the other departments should act unprofessionally toward you, do not lower yourself to that level. Report any incidents to your chief technologist and let him settle them in a diplomatic manner. Always put your best foot forward.

Cooperation with the Resident or Interne

Residents and internes, as a rule, have only a small degree of knowledge of radiographic procedures or the reading of radiograms; however, do not forget that they have put in several years of tough work and study at medical school. When they have finished their internship or their residency they will be qualified doctors of medicine and may even come on the staff of your hospital.

Any residents or internes are grateful for whatever help you can give them; they appreciate seeing interesting radiograms. In order to learn, they must see all the radiograms of the patients on their service. Remember, also, that often they are chasing you to do something the referring physicians are hounding them to do. Just because they are under the supervision of the doctors does not mean they fall in the same category that you do. They are doctors who have passed the examinations toward the "M.D." degree. You must treat them with respect as you would every physician on the staff. Usually it is quite easy to get along with internes. They are interested in explaining medical diagnoses to you in return for seeing interesting radiograms. New physicians, recently out of a university, starting to interne, may order more radiograms on a patient than may appear necessary. Do not question this, as these young people are still practicing out of the book. Later on, with experience, they will be more discreet in their requests for radiograms. At any rate, they are under the supervision of a staff doctor who will counsel them.

As a student, you can learn a great deal from internes and residents. Watch how they handle patients and learn from experience.

Young internes and residents are very often single men embarking on a serious career in life, one respected by all. With the radiology departments having a number of young, eligible, attractive female students we often run into a small problem. Overfriendliness on the part of either student technologists or the internes could prove hazardous to the position of all. Quite naturally, there are technologists who will want to meet eligible internes and perhaps marry them. Who could disbar Cupid; however, any association with the internes, outside the rules set by the Code of Ethics, can disrupt the whole department and everyone concerned.

Internes and residents quite frequently ask the radiologic technologists if they see anything significant in the radiograms. You are not qualified to read radiograms or to diagnose. Your position is to get good quality radiograms so that abnormalities may be seen, if present. Many problems arise from the above situation and after due consideration perhaps the following would be an effective solution. If the interne finds the fracture, then all is well, but if there is a fracture visible to you and he misses it, what should you do? If you do not tell him, he, no doubt, will get into trouble. Most important of all, however, the patient may receive further injury if the fracture is not properly treated. Now, if you point out the fracture, he may be outwardly thankful for your alertness, but you have dented his professional pride. He may feel quite defeated to have a minor student technologist show him—a qualified doctor—a fracture that he, himself, did not detect. Remember, *never* try to degrade the interne and feel you have raised your standards by doing so. It is human to err and you are subject to it, too. Perhaps the following means could be used to meet the situation. Remember that tact and diplomacy will take you a long way towards becoming a professional individual.

If you see that the interne is about to walk away from a radiogram which shows a fracture, start asking questions about the various images on the radiogram. First, ask him about the different processes and condyles that are normally visible. As he gets involved in explaining, eventually point to the suspected fracture area and see if he notices it. Most times he will, and his feelings will not be hurt because he detected it. If he still doesn't see it, find a normal radiogram of the same area and view and see if they compare. If they do not, ask him why and then he may investigate it clinically and detect the fracture. Do not jump to conclusions when seeing what you think appears to be a fracture —you will very often be incorrect! You can only aggravate the interne. He may hold it against you for questioning him, and, after all, what right or qualifications do you have? You will find through experience that you must think, judge, and evaluate before you voice any opinion. Everyone learns a certain amount through trial, error, and evaluation—in one word, "experience." This applies to one and all, radiologic technology student or interne.

Cooperation with the Referring Physician

One of the first questions in this section is, What does the physician expect of a radiologic technologist, particularly a student technologist? The physician may expect many qualities in a technologist but they all add up only to a few basic ones. The physician expects a technologist to be efficient and have a complete knowledge of his work. He must also be able to work with speed and accuracy to produce a quality radiogram and avoid the necessity of repeats. The technologist must show an interest and pride in his work as well as a willingness to work beyond the call of duty. The physician's prime concern is the patient; he does not consider his own comfort or convenience. He is an individual devoted to his profession and all who work with him are expected to display the same devotion to duty.

In the routine order of the day, the doctor may work calmly, almost casually. In an emergency he becomes swift and efficient; he expects all who work with him to work accordingly. He does not always have time to consider you; that is, who you are or what you are. The welfare of the patient comes first.

The question that comes to your mind is how can you help him most. Basically, your task is to produce quality radiograms as quickly as possible. Both student and graduate technologists try so hard to help sometimes, but in their excitement they are more of a hindrance. Be very careful when assisting the doctor in examining or bandaging a patient. Do only as much as he asks, no more and no less. If he does not ask for help, stand by quietly, out of his way.

Like every student and technologist, you want to win the doctor's confidence. In this, there are no short-cuts. Show him that you can get the best radiograms, in the shortest period of time, under the most adverse conditions. The doctor will appreciate an individual who can remain calm under stress and produce quality radiograms. He will respect an individual with a genuine interest in his work and in helping the patient. In this profession you do not and cannot smooth-talk your way into anything, unless its dismissal from training. When one works and deals in the health of human lives there is no room for false pretenses.

Cooperation with the Various Hospital Personnel

In summarizing this section, it would be well to remind you of the following facts. A hospital is like unto an organized community whose purpose it is to improve or restore man's health. For this organization to function properly and smoothly, all its personnel must cooperate with one another. Anyone with a personality problem causing conflict with other hospital personnel only hinders its efforts and purpose. A hospital is no place for ill-tempered, impatient individuals. If such is your problem, you must either leave training or make a drastic adjustment. This advice is for the benefit of you as well as "mostly for the patient."

CHAPTER XXIV

YOUR RESPONSIBILITY IN A DOCTOR'S OFFICE

MOST of your training will take place in an accredited institution, but many schools may have affiliated programs with clinics. Many times the radiologists in the hospital department also have a downtown office. In such a situation, students may be sent for a month or more to gain experience in a small department as well as to gain office experience. Many technologists who graduate from large institutions will go to smaller departments to work. They may seek employment in small private offices where they will be the only technologist. For the benefit of these people, some factors you should know are briefly outlined.

Mode of Dress*

Unlike the hospital, where there are several people on a staff, you will be the focus of attention the moment the patients walk into the office. The first thing they will notice is your appearance. In a private office the technologist must try to be immaculate. The uniform should be relatively simple and not "too tight," the hose white with straight seams and shoes white and clean. Do not forget to wash shoelaces. General good grooming and personal hygiene are a must. The patients would hardly wish to be cared for by some slovenly person whom they doubt would know a radiograph from a photograph. On the other hand, they might doubt the efficiency of some slinky, painted doll who looked like she would rather be in the movies. Remember to be neat, clean, and to look professional.

---

* Covered previously is a section on your method of dress, makeup, etc., to which you may wish to refer.

Greeting the Patient

Your manner of greeting the patients is of utmost importance. Remember you are representing more than just yourself. You must make the patients feel that you are pleased to see them and will do your utmost to help them, even if it is five minutes before closing time. Obtain the personal information needed before you can do the examination. Do not make the patients feel like they are a number or just a backache. Treat them as individuals important in themselves. If you are pleasant and courteous it will make the patients feel more secure to be in your care. If you are snippy and curt, and treat the patients as if they just mean more work for you then you are a failure. No one needs a technologist of this personality trait, much less in a private office.

Business Attitude

Maintain a professional attitude, be precise but do not hurry the patients or become annoyed if they have trouble supplying you with certain information. They may not remember when they were to the office last or had a radiologic examination. Older people will have a hard time remembering, as their minds work slower, so make suggestions in a pleasant manner that may remind them of something. The patients will respect you for a little bit of kindness and thoughtfulness shown.

After the initial information is obtained, you are ready to begin the examination. Give the patients gowns and sheets and show them where to change. Give a patient assistance as required. Your attitude in doing the radiography should be one of knowledge, speed and efficiency. If you carry on a pleasant conversation as the examination allows, you will make the patient's time on that hard x-ray table pass more quickly.

Doctors' offices are, as a rule, notorious for keeping patients waiting, but try to avoid this and make your schedule full but spaced to keep waiting minimized. You will see that the patients appreciate this courtesy although they may or may not tell you directly. When the radiographic examinations are complete do not leave the patients on the tables but make them comfortable in the dressing rooms. Explain to them that you will be in the darkroom developing the films so they know what you are doing. Be sure the patients know where the rest rooms are.

Before the patient leaves the office, consult your schedule and inform the patient of his next appointment or that he will be notified the date of his appointment at a later date. Be certain to explain thoroughly any instructions you may have for the patient in preparation for further examinations. Be certain to ask the patients if they have any questions and allow yourself the time to spend with them in instruction or discussion. If the patients feel that you are too busy, and anxious to get rid of them, they may feel reluctant to ask questions which may be very important to them.

Darkroom work should be as prompt as possible so that you may come out and do any repeat films that are necessary or tell the patients that they may get dressed. Try not to keep the patients waiting long, as we all tend to become restless while waiting.

Paying the Bill

While the patients are getting dressed you will be doing some of the book work, such as the billing and other entries necessary. Have the bill totaled for the patients and present it. Quite often this information may have been given you by the doctor as to the method of payment. If such is not the case, then courteously ask the patients how they wish the bill to be paid. The patients may pay in cash, by check, or some other suitable arrangement. If they have insurance, then get the number of the policy so that the office may submit the bill to the insurance company. Never throw a bill in front of a patient and say "twenty dollars please." This may be acceptable in a department store, but not in the office of a medical professional clinic. Let the patients make the plans for whatever fits their situation best and accept it in a professional manner.

When the patients prepare to leave, make them feel that it was a pleasure to serve them and that they would be welcome to come back should they be in further need of your service. Treat all patients as individuals; that is very important to them. Never deprive patients of their self-respect.

Office radiographic work depends mostly on the technologist. The radiologist will be present only for certain examinations so that the actual business promotion factor depends upon you. The efficiency, cleanliness and reputation of the department all depends on you. Whether the patients ever come back to your office should they require further work, or go somewhere else, depends mostly on you. Therefore, you must realize that the actual success of the private office is in your hands.

Most of the points mentioned with regard to office work also apply to the office in the hospital. Many training schools rotate their students to handle the office procedures such as getting information, typing reports, filing, etc. In meeting the public you must be poised, courteous, and professional. You must be able to communicate with any and every patient that comes to you. A good portion of the reputation of the department depends upon the office staff.

Perhaps you now have fully realized that no matter where you work in the department, you are on trial and under observation. Your conduct must be above reproach, your attitude and actions must be professional. Never for one moment forget that your purpose is service to your ailing fellow man. Never forget that purpose was responsible for this profession coming into being. If you have chosen radiologic technology as a profession just to please someone else or add to your own selfish self-importance, then you do not belong here. Your technical skills can be developed and improved through learning and practice but there has to be an inner desire to serve and a devotion to duty. Learn everything you can and remember it, for you may be responsible for teaching others in the near future. Each of us must contribute to our profession, not just take from it. If we are motivated by these inner ideas then we can do no less than our best and this feeling will be transmitted to our patients. They will come back to us not out of necessity but because they know we will try to help as much as we are able.

CHAPTER XXV

THE TECHNOLOGIST'S PLACE IN HIS PROFESSIONAL ORGANIZATION

EVERY professional body of people who work for a common cause, towards a common goal, must have an executive organization, established rules and regulations, and be governed thereby. It is this organization, when approved and recognized, that officially gives its members their status in society. This organized body sets the standards for qualified membership and awards diplomas or degrees accordingly.

Radiologic technologists have such an organized body, known as the American Registry of Radiologic Technologists, the purpose of which is the education of its members. This organization is made up of technologists and radiologists whose duties include setting up examinations for the graduating students as well as refresher courses and fellowship lectures for instructors, chief technologists, and administrative technologists. Your instructors will be able to give you the history of the Registry and how it was formed. It is hoped that you will realize what the Registry means to you and why it is an important organization.

The American Registry of Radiologic Technologists is an organized body which is recognized by the American Medical Association, the American College of Radiology, the American Hospital Association, and other medical societies. An individual who has trained for two years under a radiologist (a member of the American College of Radiology) in a school approved by the Registry and passes the Registry Examinations will become a Registered Radiologic Technologist. As a Registered Radiologic Technologist, this person is qualified to operate radiographic equipment owned by either a physician or medical institution. When you become a Registered Radiologic Technologist you are recognized by all of the organizations which recognize the American Registry of Radiologic Technologists.

The American Society of Radiologic Technologists is an organized body open for membership to Registered Radiologic Technologists. The Board of Directors and Officers are elected to guide the functions of the organization. Annually, national conventions are held where educational papers are presented and displays of radiograms and the latest advancements in techniques are made available for all technologists to see and study. There are business meetings at which new by-laws are presented and passed, and old laws amended for the betterment of the profession. Every organized body has a code of ethics and laws. These must be reviewed and changes made as required by the changing times. Events in the world of medicine change rapidly and the standards of our professional societies change rapidly also. We must advance our profession equally with every other medical field. Our profession is one of the newest of the paramedical fields. We still have a great deal to do to make ourselves one of the strongest organizations in the medical society. There are a number of people doing radiography without organized training, and this hinders our profession. This problem must be eradicated. The American Society of Radiologic Technologists is constantly working to elevate the educational and professional standards of the profession with the help of the American Registry of Radiologic Technologists and the American College of Radiology.

You are now enrolled in a training school accredited by the American Registry of Radiologic Technologists and the American College of Radiology. Before 1943 there was no organized system for the training of students. There was no basic curriculum or teachers' syllabus for teaching purposes in schools of radiologic technology. The training was done at random and the best possible with a minimal number of texts. Our schools now have organized libraries and follow the basic curriculum adopted by the American Society of Radiologic Technologists.

You may be wondering exactly how all this will affect you. The American Society of Radiologic Technologists is made up of the majority of the registered radiologic technologists in the country. Each state has a society which has elected officers and an executive body. Within each city or district are hospitals, private offices and clinics, all employing technologists. These technologists, in turn, make up the local or district societies. Starting then, from the smallest organized group, we have the local societies which combine to form the state societies which combine to form the American Society of Radiologic Technologists. As a student you will be eligible to be a member, to hold office and serve on various committees in your local society. You may serve on committees in your state society but you cannot vote or hold office. When you graduate and receive your Registration Diploma you will automatically become a member of the American Registry of Radiologic Technologists and eligible to become a member of the American Society of Radiologic Technologists.

At this time note that your radiologic technologist certification is only valid as long as you belong to the Registry and follow its rules, regulations, and Code of Ethics. Should you ever violate any of these rules, you can lose your certification and no longer be allowed to use the designation "R.T." after your name. Dues must be paid annually.

As a student you will wonder what you can do and where you fit in. First, join both your local and state societies. Pay your membership fees and start attending all of the local society meetings. These will be held monthly with a recess during the mid-summer months. Become interested in the various programs that will be sponsored by your local society, take advantage of what it has to offer. If there is an educational program, pay especial attention at this meeting for the material will no doubt be something very new and can be used to full advantage. If there is a fund-raising function, support it. These funds are to be used to promote the educational programs or help finance the annual state convention. Annually, there will be a two- or three-day state convention. Attend and take advantage of the unusual displays, extraordinary radiograms, essays and new equipment. You will hear many carefully chosen speakers on subjects that pertain to your studies. With this program you can only progress in your work and outlook in this professional field.

How can an organization function properly or, better yet, what is needed for it to survive? You, entering this profession, are also responsible for the professional organization. No organization or educational body can long endure if the members do not support it wholeheartedly. By supporting your society and becoming active in its functions you are indirectly raising the standards of your profession and making yourself known in the medical world. If you take advantage of the programs the society has to offer but do not support its efforts financially or through participation then you are failing in your obligations. If the local societies were to fold up, so eventually would the American Society of Radiologic Technologists and what then for the R.T.? So, you see, you are working for yourself just as much as for anyone else when you support your local society. Take advantage of all the opportunities for advancing yourself in society activities. Write essays, present displays and compete for the awards offered. Try to become a leader and if chosen as a committee chairman work with your members so that success could be the only result.

Our predecessors worked long and hard to establish our profession; as a result we have a recognized body that will award your radiologic technologist certification when you qualify. This is a young profession; there are many frontiers to be opened in the field. There are books to be written, techniques to be improved, positions to be discovered, and equipment and accessories to be modified. There is no limit to how far you can progress in this field, for, if you are an individual with ambition and foresight, you do have the opportunities. You should not stand in the background and let others do the work and worrying. You must contribute your share, even much more than you personally will benefit. You may not see the results and benefits of your efforts immediately, for it is a slow process. This attitude of determination made our country the greatest, as is true in any successful enterprise. You must maintain this attitude in your work, your studies and in supporting your local and state societies. Together we can make our profession one of the strongest and professionally qualified in the paramedical fields. By doing so we are improving the medical work in the nation and the health of its people.

The radiologic profession is no proper place for technologists who want to use it solely for the purpose of selfish benefit. How was this organized educational body formed? Do you think it was by technologists who only thought of themselves? Contrarily, they were individuals devoted to the profession, its aims and purposes!

They wanted to improve its standards and organize an educational and governing body so that the future technologists would not have the hardships their predecessors had endured. They looked into the future and could see that there was a hope for this profession. There was a need to continue to build it. There is no end to this building process and the more it grows in stature so do we. Do you want to work for the next twenty years for the same wage you started at as a new graduate? No, of course not! Do you feel you will deserve a higher income if your standard of work is not improved with the standards of the profession? You see, you are the future technologists who will carry on your profession and perhaps teach those who will follow you. The older, present pioneers will fall back as they get older; you, the youth, will carry on and improve it. If you do not, your profession will falter and weaken and even be taken over by some stronger force who will dictate to you. You will have no vote in business matters, no freedom to discuss and will only follow the rules if you wish to remain in the profession. This is unionization. We are a professional people with a Code of Ethics; we do not need a union. We need a strong, self-governing professional society.

Now, as a student, you have the opportunity to become the best technologists in the state, even in the country. You have every opportunity for the future to be an instructor, a chief technologist, president of the state society, or president of the national society. You have the opportunity to be anything you desire in your profession. Let us hope you are now aware of the unlimited rewards available to you if you "work" in your profession! Not only monetary rewards but a feeling of self-satisfaction that you have given something of yourself to your colleagues and the technologists of the future.

The preceding paragraphs have presented some points and answered some questions you may have had about where you stand in the radiologic society, what it can do for you and what you can do for the society and the profession. Certainly you must have other questions and your instructor can help you find the answers to them. Should your instructor be a little behind in some of the answers, maybe he or she is a little behind in the society! Perhaps this would be a good time for all of you to review the matter and do something about it. After you have been active in your local or state society and you see it is not progressing like it should, do not just step aside and forget about it. Find some other interested person, or persons, and together try to stimulate the other members into action. Show the other technologists why the society should be improved, why it needs to be strong and active. Become a leader yourself and you will see how the others are following you. You will see that you have accomplished something, you are an individual with a future. You will be a successful technologist and a leader in your profession. We need people of this type, but each of you must be your own motivating force.

You may find, as your interest grows in the activities of the society, so will your interest grow in your studies and your work. Through the years, a common observation is that students who are active in society work are usually the ones with high standards in their academic and practical work. These students comprise a versatile group and can handle their studies much better. This is due to the fact that they enjoy their work and are much more interested in it because of the extra activities. Such devotion is commendable and will serve as an inspiration to others.

CHAPTER XXVI

THE TECHNOLOGIST'S PLACE IN
HIS COMMUNITY

YOU may be training and working in communities of all sizes, some metropolitan, others suburban. Regardless of where you live you must realize that you will be in the public eye in your social conduct as well as within the hospital walls. Even though you do not take the hospital problems home with you, you will find that some of that proper conduct will wear off when you are off duty. This is not to imply that you are a branded lot and must walk around with "halos" above your heads, but, at the same time, you cannot be dragged out of the gutter in the morning and go to work. Somewhere you must draw the line and have some rules to live by. This line is a little higher than for the average Mr. X in the street. Perhaps Mr. X makes a little more money than you, but your profession gives you somewhat more respect and personal pride. The nature of your work and your devotion to duty make you an individual respected by the majority of the public. Your work and the work of other medical professions fall into a category of people devoted to a special kind of service to their fellow man. Not everyone or just anyone can do medical work. Medical work requires much study and practice by people of more than average intelligence. Now that we are in a position of respect by virtue of our profession, let us commence to live up to it. The public is made up of people of innumerable beliefs, ways of life, and personal opinions. Of course we can not please everyone in our public conduct but let us remember our responsibilities and please as many as we can. We must remember that even when we are off duty we represent the institution where we work. At a convention or other statewide event, it may surprise you to notice the difference in behavior of people from different institutions. The students from one institution may appear sombre and quiet, those from another may be polite and friendly. On the other hand, there may be a group of students that are loud, obscene, and drink too much, contrary to the group of people gathered. Your teaching and discipline in the department may be part of the trouble, especially if rules are lax. However, it could also be the friends you keep who influence your behavior in public.

Let us look into the problems of social drinking and your profession. Social drinking, if you are of age and it falls within the realms of your beliefs, is your own business. It is socially acceptable in all circles and walks of life. On the other hand, if you drink too much and come staggering out of a bar there will be repercussions. This conduct can only detract from the reputation of you, your department, and your profession.

In a small community, one of the two technologists at the hospital was known for the "best parties" in town! None of the people around particularly cared for this individual or the profession he represented. If they wanted a wild party or a gay time they chose him, of course, but even these same people did not want any part of him professionally. They were not willing to put themselves in his hands if they needed a radiographic examination. His parties often were comprised of many other professional people, too. In the eyes of the public what do you think was the reputation of this group of people? Do you think the public could rely on this technologist in work involving ethical confidence? To a few people this may have meant little but to the majority it meant a great deal.

A physician was known to state that his patient refused to have radiography done in a certain hospital because she had seen one of the female technologists come out of a bar with a man on each arm. This incident happened several months prior to her necessity for radiography and could have been perfectly harmless, but that was not the impression the public got. A person who drinks to excess may also quickly land in trouble with his colleagues. No one wants to associate with someone who possesses no self-control.

These are only a couple of incidents that may exemplify the problem. Alcohol loosens your inhibitions and weakens your self-control. This is undesirable in a professional person who has something important to uphold and protect.

Your private life at home is definitely your own business; at least, it should be. Your neighbors know you and where you work. If you live an average, quiet life, this is fine, but if you have a contingent of the opposite sex coming and going from your apartment, then watch out! This, plus a wild party or two, can really put your name in the number one spot in the gossip circle. Perhaps you will say you do not care what people think, but in this day of anonymous letters and telephone calls somebody will tell on you. You would not be the first to be expelled from training or employment because Mrs. Anonymous called the radiologist and asked, "did you know that so-and-so, etc.?" Do not ever place yourself in a compromising situation where people can talk about you. Ridiculous! Unfair! Defamation of character, you say; well, you are correct. Gossip is a sickness in our society but it is here to stay. When you work with the public, with matters private and confidential to it, you have to realize that it expects your character to be above reproach. It may feel that after one too many drinks you may discuss private things you know about your patients. It is not aware that we are taught to believe strongly in the value of professional ethics and professional confidence. It may judge us according to the weaknesses of others without ethical training. However, you must admit that anyone under the influence of alcohol cannot be completely trusted, no matter how thoroughly he was taught. Do not put yourself in that position.

Neither can we afford to get into any trouble with the police. Any infraction of the law will get your name in the paper; the police may telephone the institution where you are employed for information. It is quite obvious that if you become involved in anything criminal, no matter how minor, you should be dismissed from training or employment. No institution can afford to have its reputation jeopardized because of an employee who did not care enough to protect it. The hospital deals in service to the public, the commodity is the health of the public and cannot be entrusted to the hands of anyone except the most competent, skilled, and trustworthy of employees.

Physicians, nurses, and other professional persons do not strive to get their names in the papers for personal reasons. They are hard-working, skilled, trained people in honored professions but humble by virtue of these professions. Their forms of advertising are the many people they have helped to regain their health, who have returned to their homes, their jobs, and continue to function as useful citizens. We must also maintain our standards at this level. We need not fade into obscurity and not let the public know that we are trained, skilled, have an active functioning organization and are constantly striving to improve ourselves. It should be made aware that we meet regularly and seek to improve the educational programs for our students, as well as for the graduate technologists, the instructors, and those in administrative positions.

Hospitals or medical people do not advertise their services as do commercial firms. We are providing a professional service, not a product. No one comes to a certain radiology department because it was advertised that it has just set up some new equipment. Patients come to us because they are ill and in need. Their physicians send them to us. No one plans a car accident and breaks both legs just to try out our service. Patients come to us in need of service and they know we are available, but we do not need to advertise on radio or television for them to know we exist.

In discussing this matter with several people and members of the public outside the institution, one conclusion can be drawn. The general public does not particularly want us to be social butterflies always in the limelight. Due to the confidential nature of our work, experience, the human events we see daily, the public feels we should be more reserved in our public life. Even though it is mostly imagination, they fear they might be the topic of social conversation. This may sound strange to you, but you will have to accept the fact that the human mind is one of the most unpredictable and difficult devices you will encounter. It is just something we in our profession must accept and live with.

The two medical professions that the public is most familiar with are physicians and nurses. The other specialized professions with which it has a shorter contact period are less known. In passing near a hospital you will see nurses coming to and from work. You may conclude this simply because they are dressed in white uniforms, shoes and hose, with a cape or perhaps just a coat. You may see them later in a downtown store or on the street in the same attire. Ethically speaking, they should not appear in public in their uniforms, but let us now concern ourselves with our own profession.

One technologist, recalling his own experience in early training (before he had learned better), walked home one day in his uniform. Even though he wore a topcoat, part of his uniform was still visible. He was greeted by several people quite respectfully: "good afternoon, doctor"; "hello, doctor"; etc. Do you think he felt flattered? Truthfully, he felt rather foolish. If his ego had been lifted, it was lowered rather suddenly when a sweet little old lady asked if he was one of the orderlies at the hospital. Ethically, he would have been in the wrong to feel honored at being called "doctor" and continuing the parade. On the other hand, he was a student radiologic technologist and did not want to be pulled down from his level. Needless to say, this was the last time he ever wore his uniform on the street. Do not ever falsely believe you are going to raise your prestige by parading in your uniform and pretending you are someone that you really are not. It will be a shortlived pride when you see a waitress in a downtown hamburger joint wearing the exact same uniform. So, you see, you will not have gained a thing, will you? Ethically, and for sanitary reasons, the working uniform should not be worn outside the hospital. Flaunting the name of the profession you are connected with is cheap, especially if your behavior is not befitting to the profession. With this type of behavior you are putting yourselves back in the college level bracket where everyone wears a letter on his jacket. The public will have less confidence in your competence as radiologic technologists in the hospital if you act like a bunch of juveniles on the outside.

Upon talking with a number of physicians, nurses, and other people we concluded that the public is slowly losing respect for the medical profession. Many years ago the doctor was the most important of men in the community. He had prestige and was held in awe and respect because doctors were few and precious. He was on call every hour of the day, every day of the week, every week of the year. No one was ever turned away because it was after office hours. He travelled in all kinds of weather, any distance, by any means, just to reach someone in need. We do not see quite that depth of devotion today. Everything is becoming so commercialized that the whole profession is becoming more like a business. We find that the patients expect, demand, and complain more than ever and we must meet their demands. The service, care, and facilities are much more modern and effective but some of the feeling of personal service has been lost. Perhaps we, ourselves, are more responsible than anyone for this lessening of respect. What are we going to do about it? This question is difficult to answer and there are many possible solutions. Perhaps we could become less materialistic and more idealistic when we deal with our fellow man. Perhaps we could put just a little more personal feeling into our work. We must be ever mindful of our Code of Ethics and professional conduct. If we are to be respected for ourselves and our profession, we must be worthy of it!

CHAPTER XXVII

PERSONAL LIFE OF THE STUDENT
RADIOLOGIC TECHNOLOGIST

IN this democratic country we are pretty well able to do as we please in our choice of friends, our actions within the rules of society, and the law. By having young people work, study, and practice together in the hospital we will inevitably see emotional linking between some of these individuals. They may start dating and as time goes on they could become quite serious and young love will flourish.

This section has been made completely separate so that it does not get lost among all the others on personal conduct. It is hoped that you will refer to it for your own benefit.

Basically, you should try to keep your personal life, dating, etc., outside of the hospital personnel. If you start dating one of your colleagues from class you will run into many problems. First of all, no matter how discreet you are, you will find that if you work with the person you keep company with, it will be very difficult to maintain a professional atmosphere while on duty. To maintain a professional attitude towards someone you feel close to is quite a feat of self-discipline and only few can meet it. Sooner or later you will weaken and forget that you are on duty and not on a "date." This sort of behavior cannot be tolerated as it disrupts the whole department and lowers its professional standards. This daydreaming will not be tolerated or respected by the instructors or the radiologists, least of all the physicians or their patients. They will not feel free to trust anyone whose mind is off their work and up on cloud nine with Cupid.

Many tarnished tales go around about the incidents that may occur within the walls of the hospital. Other institutions, such as large industries, have many employees and frequent romances but are not subject to as much criticism. In the hospital where we deal with people rather than a product we find that the public, as a whole, expects the hospital personnel to be above reproach. For this reason hospital work is more difficult because we are more prone to criticism and always under the public eye.

If you should develop a romantic relationship with a person from another department the news will spread just that much farther and faster. No matter if your relationship is above board and proper, people tend to and will think the worse. Should gossip develop and reach the ears of your superiors or the administration, for the benefit of the institution you and your friend will likely both be dismissed. This may seem unfair but, again, the chief concern is for the hospital as a whole, and the standards of conduct it must maintain.

If you must date someone from the hospital, then curtail all your contacts to off-duty hours and outside of the hospital. Do not hold hands down the hallway or visit at each other's department so that gossip can start—and it will. Your private life is your own, so keep it private. Remember, your time on duty is for professional work and study. If you follow these rules you will find life will go along more smoothly and you will earn respect as a level-headed, serious professional individual and worthy of your profession. Know when to work, when to study, when to relax and when to enjoy your leisure time.

Social contact with the graduate staff may vary upon the policies of your particular institution. Even though you may attend the same society gatherings, departmental parties, etc., remember to maintain the same level of respect as you would while on duty. You cannot socialize on the same level and still retain a professional relationship within the hospital.

It is true that outside of the hospital the instructors have no authority over you, and rightly so. At this point, if you are not mature enough to control your emotions and behavior, then you are not mature enough to remain in training for the profession of radiologic technology.

Relative to romantic involvement of students and graduate technologists, it is difficult to clearly define rules for such a situation. Surely this is not recommended policy. This could place the student in question at a disadvantage with the other students.

These students would be inclined to feel that this student would enjoy advantages they were not at liberty to use. On the other hand, the graduate in question may be isolated by his colleagues, thus also creating a problem. It is hoped to point out that there are no benefits as far as the profession, the department, or the institution are concerned. There is no personal advantage as far as furthering your training is concerned.

As student technologists you will be required to attend many local and state meetings and associated functions. It is quite common to see students indulging in careless, youthful, exuberant behavior at these functions. It never seems to fail that some of them will gain access to alcoholic beverages (even if they are not of age), overindulge, and end up behaving rather shamefully. Such behavior is a discredit to the school and the profession. If you are of age, and have the right to drink, this is acceptable, but for any student to reach the state of insensibility and loss of self-control must demonstrate a form of weakness of character. A student, who is a minor, becoming intoxicated at a professional gathering and later becoming involved in a traffic mishap could create quite a problem for the society in question. The parents of the student may refuse to accept responsibility and the sponsors of the function would be liable for a lawsuit, for contributing to the delinquency of a minor.

In summary, exercise self-restraint, indulge in a little common sense, set a code of moral and ethical conduct personally and professionally, and adhere to it.

SUMMARY

WHAT I HOPE YOU HAVE LEARNED

Now that you are at the end of this book, the author hopes that your mind is full of thoughts and just as full of questions. His desire for this book is that it should motivate your thinking. You should have learned something, but, on the other hand, you may disagree with some of the statements. If you do, then you have become conscious of the problems discussed and have a healthy attitude. This means that you can think for yourself.

By now you should have realized the necessity of ethics and professional conduct in your work. You should be conscious of the fact that in each day of your training and in later work you will be faced with problems. Any errors you make, no matter how small and insignificant they may seem to you, look much different in the eyes of the public, and the patients. And, of course, in your line of work, the patients, their comfort and their welfare are your prime concern. Any small errors you may make may cause them worry, may become magnified and intensified to them just because you did not have the foresight to prevent them. These patients may feel they were not treated properly or were abused psychologically.

Just sit back a few moments and think about the problems you unconsciously create in your work and never realize it. Do not ever be foolish enough to believe that these errors could not happen to you personally; if you have already worked with patients, you will have realized it by now. Do not think that you can shrug these matters off and pretend they did not happen.

When you come in contact with numerous people day after day you must learn to be flexible and adapt yourselves to every personality. You must always maintain your composure and professional dignity. If you have radiographed patients in the early part of your training you will have realized that it is not as easy as it looked when you watched the seniors do it. You have watched them handle patients with skilled, learned manners. This was accomplished only through study and practice, often learned the hard way. You must understand that people have many peculiarities and differences in personality to which you must become accustomed. You must try never to give them any reason to doubt or complain about you. You must make them feel that you are a learned, competent, professional person and they must feel secure in your care.

As you read all the material in this book it should have motivated you to improve your conduct, expanded your knowledge and given you ideals on how to improve yourself. If so, you will be a benefit to the patient, the profession, and to yourself. Many books may be written on this subject and you may read them all but none of them will do you any good if you do not think about the material and try to apply it. You must be able to criticize yourself and see where you have failed. Every student must realize that just doing good radiography is not the true answer to the qualities of a top rated radiologic technologist. In a recent survey by an independent organization on why people lose their positions in any field of employment, it was discovered that 35 per cent was due to lack of knowledge and 65 per cent to personality problems and conduct.

After some years of teaching and being active in radiographic work, the author wishes to tell you that he often sits back and thinks about many small problems of ethics and conduct that seem to have been passed over. Every problem, be it large or small, is important to the patient-technologist relationship. This relationship must be improved with each succeeding generation of technologists.

It may seem very difficult at first for a high school graduate or college boy or girl to step into a world of sickness and disease, to be in constant contact with people who are worried, afraid, unhappy and just generally miserable.

It is a grim world where a person must have stamina, ambition, and devotion to duty in order to be a success. Perhaps, in some small way, this book may contribute to your success. We need more professionally dedicated people; will you be one of these?

The X-Ray Technician's Pledge

I solemnly pledge that I will cheerfully and willingly assist the Radiologist in all diagnostic and therapeutic Radiological Procedures to the best of my ability.

I will procure the best possible films in all examinations.

I will treat every patient with courtesy and consideration.

I will take care to maintain a professional attitude in my relationship with all patients.

I will regard as strictly confidential all information regarding each patient coming for examination or treatment.

I will not discuss patients nor their affairs outside of the X-Ray Department. I will not divulge to the patient the results of any examination.

I will do all in my power to live up to and to improve the highest traditions of my profession.

So help me, God!

Code of Ethics

Applicants for certification in radiation therapy technology must, at the time of application, and on subsequent occasions when the certificate is renewed, agree to abide by the following code of ethics:

"In consideration of the granting to me of a certificate of registration, or the renewal thereof, and the attendant right to use the title "Registered Radiation Therapy Technologist" and its abbreviation, "R.T. (ARRT)", in connection with my name, I do hereby agree to perform the duties of a radiation therapy technologist only under the supervision of a person whose qualifications are acceptable to this Registry; and to abide by all the rules and regulations of The American Registry of Radiologic Technologists as they apply to my profession; and to conduct myself in a manner appropriate to the dignity of my profession consistent with the Principles of Medical Ethics of the American Medical Association."

Code of Ethics

Applicants for certification in nuclear medicine technology must, at the time of application, and on subsequent occasions when the certificate is renewed, agree to abide by the following code of ethics:

"In consideration of the granting to me of a certificate of registration, or the renewal thereof, and the attendant right to use the title "Registered Nuclear Medicine Technologist" and its abbreviation, "R.T. (ARRT)," in connection with my name, I do hereby agree to perform the duties of a nuclear medicine technologist only under the supervision of a person whose qualifications are acceptable to this Registry; and to abide by all the rules and regulations of The American Registry of Radiologic Technologists as they apply to my profession; and to conduct myself in a manner consistent with the Principles of Medical Ethics of the American Medical Association."

Code of Ethics

Applicants for certification in x-ray technology must, at the time of application, and on subsequent occasions when the certificate is renewed, agree to abide by the following code of ethics:

"In consideration of the granting to me of a certificate of registration or a renewal thereof, by The American Registry of Radiologic Technologists, and the attendant right to use the title "Registered X-Ray Technologist" and its abbreviation "R. T." (ARRT) in connection with my name, I do agree to perform the duties of an x-ray technologist whether as a worker, teacher or supervisor, only under the direction or supervision of a duly qualified physician.

I will not act as owner, co-owner, advisor or employer in connection with any type of enterprise having anything to do with the medical use of ionizing radiation unless it be as an affiliated registered technologist and subject to the limitations of such certification. I will not interpret radiographs or fluoroscopic shadows, treat or advise patients as to x-ray diagnosis or treatment; nor will I teach students in x-ray technology unless under the direct supervision of a duly qualified doctor of medicine who specializes in radiology; and I will abide by this code of ethics, and all other present and future rules and regulations of The American Registry of Radiologic Technologists as long as I retain my certificate."

INDEX